A Woman's Hormonal Health Survival Guide

How to Prevent Your Doctor From Slowly Killing You

DR. ANGELA DEROSA, DO, MBA, CPE

Printed in the United States of

America First Printing, 2018

SECOND EDITION
ISBN 978-0-578-40505-6 (ePub)

Publisher: DeRosa Media, LLC
11445 E. Via Linda Drive, Ste -
206 Scottsdale, AZ 85259

For more information, visit DrHotFlash.com

Edited by: Linda Williams, The Brand Counselors
Cover design and interior design: Kurt Krause, Krause Creative

Digital book(s) (epub and mobi) produced by Booknook.biz.

DISCLAIMER

While this book is intended to provide accurate and authoritative information with regard to the subject matter covered, it is not intended to provide personalized medical advice. This book should be used only as a general guide. Since the advice and strategies herein may not be suitable for your situation, you should consult a professional where appropriate. Neither the publisher nor author shall be liable for any loss, damage, or expense of any nature caused or alleged to have been caused directly or indirectly by the information contained in this book. If any health, psychological or any other expert assistance is required or appropriate, the services of a competent professional should be sought.

CONTENTS

DEDICATION

This book is dedicated to the memory of my mother and my sister. I miss you both, and I hope that I make you proud. To all the women who deserve better treatment, unbiased health information and true equality: We are women, hear us roar! We are women. We cannot and will not be ignored.

Doctors pour drugs of which they know little, to cure diseases of which they know less, into patients of whom they know nothing.

- Molière

ACKNOWLEDGEMENTS

As I sit down to think about all of the wonderful friends, colleagues and mentors that I need to acknowledge and thank for making this book a reality, I know it's likely that I will forget someone who should be included, and I apologize in advance for any oversights.

I have faced many challenges in my life, but every step of the way, I have been gifted with wonderful mentors, friends and people who have motivated me to "step up and commit to making a difference" and never, ever quit.

While I was growing up, every single day my dad pushed me to be better than I thought I could ever be. This often made me angry, but he never stopped challenging me to be exceptional. He often reminded me to never forget that the best investment I could make in life was the one I could make in myself. His advice became particularly valuable as I started down the road to medical school. Knowing that my dream of being a doctor meant I would come out on the other side saddled with close to $200,000 in debt was terrifying. Dad told me to never allow myself to be held back by fear, and made me realize it would all be OK. Dad (AKA BK), you are my hero.

It's an incredible blessing to be surrounded by many female mentors and friends. Each has inspired me to continue my quest to change the face of health care, and to hold fast to what my dream could mean for women everywhere. While I was still in high school, my guidance counselor helped me learn to believe in myself, and a dear family friend gave me the confidence I needed to pursue my goals. Jan and Cathy... you started this journey for me. God help us all.

When I decided to get onto the fast track and create a new women's health program during my internal medicine residency program at Lutheran General Hospital in Park Ridge, Illinois, I was met with resistance from directors of hospital medical departments and other physicians. They were threatened by what

I was trying to do, as well as concerned that I would "step on their clinical turf" and take patients from them. I'm forever grateful to Dr. Edward Linn, the director of the hospital's OB/GYN program, who helped me face the politics head on and encouraged me to learn all that I could about the gynecologic view of women's health. He was tough, fair and fearless. Most of all, he went out on a limb for me and I will never forget this.

During my time in big pharma, I met so many wonderful women's health providers who were living my dream of the clinical practice focused on women, and I soaked up all the knowledge and inspiration I could from them. Eventually they urged me to take the leap and open my own practice – another terrifyingly huge step. In 2010, I finally JUMPED off the cliff and opened DeRosa Medical. The foundation for making my dream of leaving a legacy in women's health became a reality.

The first few years of establishing and growing my practice have been tough and exhilarating at the same time, and I've used them to fuel my personal fire to change the face of women's health care. I continue to be blessed by the presence of a number of strong, passionate women in my life. I have deliberately surrounded myself with women who are all smart, talented, inspired, and like me, on a mission.

During my MBA program, I learned that the best way to look and be smart is to surround yourself with people smarter than you, and listen to them. I took this advice very seriously. To my circle of colleagues and friends … thank you for being my smarter circle of influence.

To Virginia Kelley: Your help in maintaining my sanity (well, most of it) and your guidance as I navigated through some of the hardest years of my life has been invaluable. Thank you.

My profound thanks goes out to my colleagues in my office (providers, clinical assistants and administrative staff) for helping me bring my vision to light every single day. Being surrounded by such positive energy and compassion I am continually inspired to do more and more in medicine and be a better doctor.

To Cyd, my best friend: you challenge me to be a better person and give me the love and attention I need to survive life's struggles and hurdles: I don't know what I did in life before you.

To Linda, my Chief Operations Officer: thank you for keeping me grounded when I find myself feeling overwhelmed, compromised or challenged in life, all while managing the three ring circus that is our medical practice. You are so wise, and have a tremendously amazing gift for dealing with people while always keeping a smile on your face and compassion in your heart.

To Kendra, my surrogate sister not only in life but medicine: You remind me of what brought me to medicine in the first place and you continue to motivate and challenge me. Your growth in medicine gives me confidence that when I am older, society will be in good medical hands.

To Anna: We always find laughter, even amongst the tears. You know where all the bodies are buried, and of course, we have our table reserved in hell. Na Zdorovie!

To Teri, my publicist: you are fierce in your passion and execution of helping me elevate my mission and without you I would be a messenger without a platform. You do so, while making me laugh, keeping me grounded and providing adequate wine when required.

My love, respect and sincere gratitude go out to each of you!
Angela DeRosa, October 20, 2018

FOREWORD

In 2014, I published this book in the hopes that I could arm women with the proper knowledge to become advocates and fierce defenders of their own health and sanity. Although this book resonated with woman of all ages, it unintentionally offended many of my colleagues. Most of them didn't even read the book; they just didn't like the title.

As I received feedback from readers, "like-minded" physicians and other medical professionals who took the time to read my book, I realized that they wanted to learn more but also wanted sound resources to do so. In addition, many women who read the book, wanted to know if I was aware of any physicians in their local communities who specialized in hormone replacement therapies. Unfortunately, the answer was often "no." There simply are not many physicians who are properly trained to care for the unique hormonal needs of women.

As a result of this feedback and knowledge, I have evolved my thinking and mission to become part of the solution. I now want to continue to ardently educate not only women directly, but also the providers who care for them. I want to educate and inspire an army of medical professionals who can help change the paradigm of women's hormonal health.

Notably, I have been asked to speak at the largest international conference of anti-aging physicians, The American Academy of Anti-Aging Medicine (A4M), to specifically address physicians and other medical professionals who want to learn more and evolve their practices regarding women's hormonal health (edited). Importantly and specifically, garnered by my decades of education and experience, I have developed a training program for physicians and other medical care providers to learn from me directly; how to incorporate bio-identical hormone therapy (BHRT) into their medical practices.

I am now focusing my time on simultaneously educating the public and medical professionals with the goal of delivering optimal hormonal healthcare for women across the United States.

In the closing chapter of my book, "Steps You Can Take Today," I will give you actionable steps you can take to join the mission in spreading the word on the powerful benefits of BHRT and the life-changing role it plays in women's health and wellness. We are in the fight for our lives, and may this hormonal health survival guide give you the power to change YOUR life...today!

INTRODUCTION

A Calling, Not a Career

When I was eight years old, I knew I wanted to be a doctor. I was good in school, liked to learn, and my parents encouraged me. I was also a born ham. Speaking or performing in public was never intimidating for me – I loved it. I adored music, too. It was fun and gave me confidence, but I never once forgot that I wanted to be a doctor. I had a mission in life, and I was driven to accomplish it. There was no second choice. So for me, medicine is a calling, rather than a career.

At the age of 12, my calling was sealed. I visited the Chicago Museum of Science and Industry, and walked through the chambers of a gigantic model of a human heart and read information on how it works. It was the coolest thing I had ever seen. I was going to be a doctor.

Music came to me as naturally as my knowledge that I was going to become a doctor, so until I could actually become a doctor, I studied hard and competed in talent competitions, playing piano and organ. Soon enough, graduation was on the horizon, and it became clear that I couldn't afford to go away to a fancy college, but there was no way I was going to give up my dream. I just had to figure out a way to make it come true.

My guidance counselor, one of my greatest mentors in life, encouraged me to begin college while I was a senior in high school, so I got a head start and saved some money that way.

I lived at home in Troy, Michigan, a suburb of Detroit, and commuted to the nearest state college, Wayne State University, located in a gritty area of downtown Detroit. I had grown up playing piano, and music helped me realize my dreams. To help pay my tuition, I worked as a private tutor, teaching piano and organ lessons in people's homes. I commuted to WSU for the remainder of my undergraduate degree and in 1990 I received a bachelor of arts in liberal arts with honors in biological sciences. I was then accepted at the Chicago College of Osteopathic Medicine in Downers Grove, Illinois. I was on my way!

I met my first husband while I was in my second year of medical school and he was in his fourth. By the time I completed my residency in Internal Medicine, we were divorced. While I didn't know it at the time, during our entire relationship I was in the middle of perimenopause and becoming hormonally deficient. It was a major factor in the breakdown and erosion of our marriage, and ultimately ignited my passion and put my career onto the path towards fulfilling my destiny of helping women.

You're Too Young to Have Hormonal Issues

I wasn't feeling great, and I most definitely wasn't feeling like me. The music of my life seemed to be missing notes, so everything was discordant and off key. I was moody and tired all the time. I didn't want to have sex. I was anxious and bordering on depression. My heart would race with palpitations, and I was put on beta blockers to slow it down. While I was still doing well academically and professionally, I was struggling to retain information – it didn't seem as easy as it once normally did.

Understandably, it was easy for me to believe these issues stemmed from the pressures of working 36-hour shifts, so I blamed everything on my residency. Looking back now, I realize I also had hot flashes and night sweats – all the typical symptoms of starting menopause. But I was only in my twenties, so how could that even be possible?

Meanwhile, I was on birth control pills, which I had no idea were making things worse for me physically, because they also provided just enough estrogen to prevent full-blown symptoms.

I was trying to figure out what was happening to me. I had a hunch it was hormonal, but I just couldn't put my finger on it. At the time, there were only 17 women's health programs in the nation. I wanted to learn more about hormones and the roles they played in women's health, so I approached Dr Marc Fine, my residency program director, about establishing a new program.

Once my idea was approved, I created all my own electives and with it, my own fast-track women's health program within the internal medicine program at Lutheran General. I worked with breast surgeons, gynecologists and others to hone in on women's health topics.

Meanwhile, as a resident, the majority of patients I was treating were female because they wanted female physicians. While many women become OB-GYNs, pediatricians, or family practice doctors, not as many choose internal medicine. Many women prefer to see a woman doctor because they assume we understand them better, which isn't always the case. Medically speaking, I wanted to learn as much as I could about what made women different so I could learn how to treat them more effectively.

Honestly, it was frustrating. Internal medicine doctors treat a lot of people who are already suffering from chronic diseases, so we feel like we make little headway. I knew there had to be a better way to do things, and I was determined to figure out how. If I could just understand where things begin to go wrong, I could then intervene and try to improve the lives of patients earlier; before they were too far beyond help, or even prevent disease from developing.

Luckily, I met a lot of people during my residency with a passion for women's health. I learned from a number of doctors who were essential to my continuing education and growth, and who motivated me to pursue women's health issues as a specialty.

Ironically, while I was busy learning everything I could about medicine, as well as hormones and how they worked, I began premature menopause – which is the onset of menopause before age 40. Premature menopause affects 10 to 20 percent of women, and causes can include genetic makeup, diabetes, lupus, medications, and environmental factors, just to name a few. However, I was never able to pinpoint the exact cause of my condition. By age 35, I hadn't had a period for over a year. I had officially reached menopause.

Forging a Pathway

By the time I graduated my residency, I was newly divorced, and in charge of the Lutheran General Hospital department I had first proposed and created during my residency, the Women's Health Education and Services Department. It was my job to open a comprehensive women's health clinic, and enhance and develop it by educating the residents coming up behind me. Preparing others to follow in my footsteps would ensure that the clinic could continue to thrive if I decided to leave my position. Eventually, I did.

While inside the hospital I was the director in charge of a fledgling women's health program, the outside world began to take notice. I was one of 12 doctors chosen to sit on an advisory panel for a new osteoporosis drug being developed by Procter & Gamble and Aventis. Being chosen for the panel was a huge step forward in my career.

I never thought I'd leave clinical practice and defect to the "dark side" of medicine, but soon enough, pharmaceutical companies began courting me to come to work on new medicines specific to women's health.

In 2000, when Procter & Gamble was ready to launch the osteoporosis drug, they recruited me to become the senior medical director of the West Coast. I wasn't happy working for "the man" at the hospital anymore, but I also had nearly $200,000 in student debt to consider. The job offer doubled my salary, the weather was better, and it was an all-around great opportunity. I happily took the job. My main responsibility was to launch the osteoporosis drug – so my initial goal was to learn everything I could about osteoporosis.

During my eight years with Procter & Gamble, I was truly excited about another project we were working on: Intrinsa, a testosterone patch for women. My job was to educate the scientific staff about female physiology and hormones and to advise the launch. In 2006, one month before the approval was to be issued, the FDA decided it wasn't safe for women and wouldn't approve it. Mind you, it was approved for use in Europe and Australia. This was American politics at its worst, and once again women and their health was on the losing side of the equation. Procter & Gamble cut back on the program, and I was no longer as interested in working there. Time for the next step forward!

Over my professional career, I'd met top experts in the women's health field. I began seriously considering starting my own clinical practice. While deciding what to do, I took two other leadership positions – first at American Physicians Inc., and later at MatrixMedical Network, where I made more great contacts.

I wanted my own practice because so few physicians focus on working in the area of women's hormones, and yet they are such an essential component of women's health. Conventional wisdom about hormones drives most of medicine, and most of it's completely wrong. Since my mission in life is to help women feel better and live better, in October 2009, I decided it was time to go for it. To fund my new practice, I maxed out all of my credit cards and jumped off the proverbial financial cliff. DeRosa Medical opened on Jan. 4, 2010.

Rattling Cages and Challenging Convention

You're probably wondering why I've decided to write a book called *"A Women's Hormonal Health Survival Guide: How to Prevent Your Doctor From Slowly Killing You,"* that's guaranteed to anger a large portion of the medical community. Simple. As a woman and a physician, I am angry. Hormone deficiencies are not limited to the realm of the menopausal, and there is no doubt in my mind we're all in a fight for our lives.

My personal and professional journey has proven time and again that women are getting bad information about hormones and hormone replacement therapy from their doctors, from the media and from the government, and it's causing a health epidemic. It's not because other doctors are sinister or incompetent – although I could certainly name more than a few of both types, most doctors are simply misinformed. Unfortunately, there are others jumping into hormone replacement therapy without understanding how hormones really work in the body, and as a result, they're making women (and men) sicker.

The most common thing I hear from patients in my practice is "Why have my other doctors missed this?" Every day there are women in my office crying grateful tears that they've found a doctor that actually listens to them; one who is determined to get to the source of the problem. They're tired of hearing that they're just stressed out or depressed, and of doctors pushing prescriptions designed to treat symptoms. It's gratifying to be able to reassure these women that they're not crazy or misunderstood, and that we have the knowledge and the tools to help them. It's called bio-identical hormone replacement therapy, or BHRT.

Educating and Empowering Women

When I first opened DeRosa Medical, we were treating women almost exclusively. Today our patient mix is closer to 60% women and 40% men. (As a women's hormonal health specialist, I get a little giggle from that stat. I promise you'll understand why when you read the first chapter.) Patients regularly travel to my practice from Alaska, Hawaii, the East Coast and even Germany to be evaluated and treated.

No matter how hard I work, I can only treat a finite number of patients, but through this book I can educate an infinite number of people. It's meant as a tool to help women of all ages understand some of the most common and commonly misdiagnosed hormonal health issues, and to arm them with the facts about bio-identical hormone replacement. Many chapters include composite case studies of patients, so readers suffering in similar ways can recognize their own symptoms, and see how others regained their health and vitality.

This book is not meant as a replacement for your doctor's advice or treatment, but as a supplemental learning tool to help you take charge of your own health. The health survival guide checklist can help women ask their provider the right questions, make sure they are getting the right tests and that their doctor is interpreting results correctly. This book was calling out to be written, and I know it can make a difference. I hope it does for you.

CHAPTER ONE

HORMONES: WHAT THEY ARE, WHAT DO THEY DO, WHY WE SHOULD REPLACE THEM

If you're a woman and feeling run down, tired and forgetful, gaining weight or experiencing any number of the symptoms of menopause, chances are you haven't had much sympathy from your doctors, let alone solutions. They'll pat you on the head and tell you nothing's wrong; saying that it's all just part of aging. Feeling achy? "Take Tylenol." Not in the mood for sex? "Schedule a date night." Getting forgetful? "We call that CRS disease - Can't Remember Shit." Gaining weight? "Get more exercise and eat healthier."

These types of responses do nothing to help us, and frankly, make women feel even worse. The underlying message is that we're to blame because we're not doing enough, and we should stop whining and simply accept feeling awful. The demands on our time and attention are already endless, and now we're supposed to do more? Many women already work eight or more hours a day, commute, run the kids around, grocery shop, cook dinner, do laundry, keep track of bills and finances, and deal with all of the daily dramas: The "check engine" light is on! The cat threw up! The toilet overflowed! The air conditioner is broken! Where's my red shirt? Mom, I need 48 cupcakes for the bake sale tomorrow, and they can't be from the store!

No wonder we're exhausted. Now we're also supposed to believe that because we eat poorly, feel worse, look rundown and have no sex life, it's our fault? I'm here to say the answer to that is "Hell, no!" Hormonal deficiencies are usually to blame.

By now, you're probably wondering what hormonal deficiencies actually are and why you should care about them. Get comfortable, and together we'll find out.

The "big three" hormones are estrogen, testosterone and thyroid, or what I call "the Axis of Evil," to borrow a phrase used by President George W. Bush. They're either with us or against us, and as we get older, they usually start to work against us.

When working properly, a woman's body makes 60 percent estrogen and 40 percent testosterone (See? There's that 60/40 ratio again.) Working properly, a man's body makes 95 percent testosterone and 5 percent estrogen. Ahem. This obviously shows that women are more balanced, much to the disbelief of the male half of the species.

As we age, both estrogen and testosterone decline, but testosterone will deplete more rapidly because:

1. We have less of it to begin with.
2. It doesn't store in the body's fat cells, like estrogen does.

In the United States the average age for menopause is 52, but this simply refers to the state when the ovaries fully retire and our periods end. All systems are down and permanently out of business. By the year 2025, it's expected that 1.1 billion women worldwide (yes, that's billion with a "B") will be in menopause. However, women enter a state of perimenopause, meaning "around menopause," 10 to 15 years before actual menopause, and that's where the trouble starts.

The Rise of the Axis of Evil

Women in perimenopause will experience three stages of hormone deficiency: testosterone deficiency and estrogen deficiency (perimenopause), and then, menopause. Keep in mind that if you talk to doctors or look this up in a medical textbook, the actual terminology is much more complicated. For the sake of simplicity, here is a breakdown of the main symptoms and differences among the stages.

Testosterone Deficiency

The hallmarks of testosterone deficiency include low libido, weight gain, low libido, anxiety, low libido, depression, and did I mention lowlibido? You may also experience mood swings, memory loss, sugar cravings and a "beer belly" appearance from the weight gain. Our shapely curves take a turn in the wrong direction. Instead of carrying our weight in our thighs, it moves to our belly. This usually starts in the mid- to late-30s, but certain medications, illnesses and genetics can cause it to begin sooner.

Estrogen Deficiency or Perimenopause (Early, mid and late stages)

During the early stage of estrogen deficiency, many women will experience hot flashes and insomnia right before and during their period. Premenstrual syndrome (PMS) gets worse, and you may have migraines for the first time in your life.

The mid stage of estrogen deficiency sees the onset of hot flashes during random times throughout month (not just during periods), worsening PMS (just when we thought it couldn't possibly get any worse), insomnia, forgetfulness and night sweats.

The late stage is usually marked by irregularity in menstrual cycles, and oh yes, worsening symptoms overall. You might go several months without getting a period (things are looking up), but suddenly, Aunt Flo is back with a vengeance, often becoming heavier and lasting longer (spoke too soon). Worse yet, your periods may become more frequent and have all of the delightful hallmarks outlined in the previous sentence. Terrific.

What About Progesterone?

You also need progesterone to prepare your body for pregnancy and to help you have regular periods. Progesterone is the controlling hormone that causes worsening PMS symptoms, and this hormone is produced after ovulation by the follicle remnants. However, if you don't make enough estrogen – which happens when your ovaries slow down – then you won't have enough progesterone, either. This leads to an estrogen dominant state, meaning the estrogen level is higher than the progesterone

3

level. You won't ovulate due to the low estrogen, and your periods get irregular. This usually begins in the early to mid-40s, but again, certain factors can trigger it to start earlier.

Welcome to Menopause (at last)

In our lifetimes, we only have a certain number of eggs in our ovaries, and when they're gone, they're gone. The age of menopause can vary, but ask your mother when she went through it, as the timeline tends to run in families. You will know you're there when you haven't had a period for more than 12 months. Although you may still be experiencing some of the unpleasant symptoms like hot flashes, insomnia and forgetfulness, along with a few new ones, at least you're not bleeding all the time. While there are blood tests (follicle stimulating hormone, or FSH, and anti-mullerian hormone levels) we can use to verify it, that's the main marker.

Thyroid: The Wild Card

The other big hormone in play is the thyroid. The thyroid is a small, bow tie-shaped organ located at the front and middle of the neck that secretes the thyroid hormone thyroxine, or T4. It converts to the active thyroid hormone triiodothyronine, or T3, at the direction of the brain. These thyroid hormones fuel and control your metabolism overall.

Imagine your thyroid as the engine of your body. Ideally, we want to be in a BMW, Lexus or Mercedes, not in a Formula One car or a go-kart.

A Formula One thyroid is hyperthyroid, and is burning fuel too fast. Everything in the body is on overdrive. This leads to weight loss, hair loss, diarrhea, high temperatures and excessive sweating.

A go-kart thyroid, or hypothyroid, is too slow. This causes weight gain, dry skin, constipation, hair loss, low body temperature, slow heart rate, extreme fatigue and swelling or numbness of hands and/or feet.

The BMW/Lexus/Mercedes thyroid, like a finely tuned machine, is running just right. Women with normal thyroid function have appropriate energy levels and feel good, assuming they have no other health issues. Their bodies are firing on all cylinders.

But here's the kicker: by the age of 50, one in three women will have a thyroid disorder; most commonly, they'll be hypothyroid. It can be caused from the aging process, autoimmune disorder, environmental factors or a combination. (We'll cover this in more depth later.)

The Axis of Evil Takes Control

Now imagine having a combination of hormone deficiencies, and low testosterone and low estrogen have decided to team up with hypothyroidism. Your whole body is working against you. The Axis of Evil has risen to power, conquered your republic, and is now soundly kicking your ass.

Now we're not only unhappy and feeling physically crappy, our body image, mental health, psychological health and overall energy levels are also impacted. Collectively, the Axis of Evil is sapping our basic ability to cope with life. Again, all too often our doctors are telling us it's all in our heads. It's not.

Hell Slowly Begins to Break Loose

With all our body systems breaking down, it's inevitable that everything going on begins to spill over into our relationships, and the most adversely affected is our love life. This is pretty important stuff. Let's hear from Virginia Kelley, a licensed clinical social worker who specializes in relationships and intimacy:

> *"Simply stated, couples who are the happiest tend to be those with good sex lives. Sexual intimacy allows us to experience closeness, vulnerability and sharing with our partner. Humans have a general desire to belong, to love and feel loved, which is usually satisfied in physically and emotionally intimate relationships. Sexual intimacy eases life's tensions. Once you start paying attention to your sexual relationship, your partner will be happier. As a result you'll enjoy being around them more so you're happier."*

5

Sadly, when there is little or no appetite for sexual intimacy by one partner, the relationship becomes more vulnerable to extramarital affairs. Most affairs occur out of opportunity. For example, if your partner would like more of a sexual relationship, and then finds an attentive and interested party, you may have the awful experience of finding infidelity in your relationship. Infidelity is very, very difficult to overcome. Rebuilding trust and recommitting to the relationship can't always be done. The hurt and pain is miserable on both sides.

Another aspect of the lack of physical intimacy is that partners in relationships will tend to become more and more distant. Communication decreases and in turn, conflicts increase, further draining your relationship. You stop being an intimate team and become the "Bickering Bickersons" or worse, two people who simply happen to live together.

When one partner is hesitant, ambivalent or not "in the mood," it's harder to have a caring and loving sexual experience (which doesn't need to be a sex romp for hours), but if you continue to do so, you'll feel better about yourselves and each other.

I asked Virginia to share a specific example of a relationship that fell apart due to lack of intimacy. Here is a case study:

> *"I recall a couple I'll call Alyssa and Jim. They were in their early fifties, had no children, and great careers. Alyssa and Jim were very physically fit and enjoyed multiple outdoor activities together. They supported each other's careers and were best friends. But they had very little sexual intimacy.*
>
> *Alyssa hadn't felt any sexual interest for about five years. Despite that, everything seemed fine between them until Jim had an affair and left Alyssa. He later told her that her lack of interest in him sexually made him feel inadequate and unattractive. Alyssa complained that he never communicated how important this was to him. Jim said he tried to ignore it until, of course, another woman made him feel sexually desirable. This is one scenario that probably could have turned out differently had they addressed the issue of lack of intimacy."*

The lack of libido, and the resulting lack of intimacy can be a relationship killer. Virginia continues:

> "Other typical cases are couples that come in for marital counseling and all they can do is argue and find fault with each other. When I ask them about their sexual relationship they admit that they rarely have time for intimacy, or are not interested and haven't been for years. When we begin to unravel the history of their relationship, we find that as their sexual intimacy waned, their arguing and complaining increased. Once again they could have changed the course of their marriage had they been able to communicate with each other the need to be physically close. Or, for that matter, even been aware of how important it was to them."

Now, we get to the physical, hormone-heavy part of the equation, which used to be the "hot and heavy" part. I asked Virginia if perimenopause or menopause makes things worse:

> "I have seen many couples in trouble with their relationship for various reasons, including lack of sexual intimacy due to perimenopause/menopause. Typically, the female is either afraid of hormone replacement or is on an incorrect HRT regimen which is not helping her with libido. So they give up and take the route of living like roommates. The husband usually speaks of his wife's irritability, mood swings and lack of ability to enjoy sex. The wife speaks of feeling unattractive, having little or no interest in sex and/or painful intercourse. So they avoid the whole issue and continue a less than satisfying marriage, believing that this is an avoidable part of aging. This, of course, does not have to be how we end our golden years!"

Amen, sister! Hormone replacement therapy (HRT) not only improves a host of age-related issues, it can also help save relationships and restore sex lives.

HRT: Not Just for Menopause Anymore

Some of you are probably thinking, "Wait. Isn't menopause just a natural state of aging that all women go through? Why fight it?" My answer is this: Yes, it's natural and if we live long enough, we'll all go through it. But think about it this way: Not all that long ago in the scheme of history, fewer women lived to see menopause because so many didn't survive their vulnerable childbearing years. Men who didn't die fighting some war or another would soldier on, often remarrying and fathering children well into their old age.

Women died before, during and after childbirth due to complications and infections. They died from sexual violence, misinformation, misogyny and political or religion-fueled madness. Women and young girls were accused of witchcraft, and then drowned or burned at the stake. Yes, menstrual cycles and fluctuating hormone levels can make us feel pretty witchy, but c'mon guys!

However, karma has a way of coming around. While hormone imbalances can occur at almost any age, today most women can expect to live anywhere from one third to one half of their lives in menopause; so of course we want these years to be healthy, happy and fulfilled. HRT can help us achieve it, so why is it so hard to get?

Unfortunately, when it comes to women and their health and reproductive issues, misinformation and misogyny continue to be dominant forces, along with political or religion-fueled madness. And money. Oh, so much money. It's well past the time that we start taking control of the conversation and of our own health, or women will continue to be dismissed.

CHAPTER TWO

CHALLENGES, MYTHS AND MISCONCEPTIONS ABOUT HRT

So if hormone deficiencies are ruining women's health, lives and love lives, why aren't doctors doing something about it? Oh, you can bet there's a big laundry list of reasons, and most of them are going to make you just as irritable as hormone deficiencies can. Let's take a look at the major issues.

Politics Versus Facts

There's still a huge gender bias in our culture and in medicine. It's the 21st century, and women's sexuality continues to be a topic of controversy. Today, we have an overwhelming number of men (and even women) in Congress and State government who want to legislate control of women's bodies. We're still having arguments about contraception and reproductive healthcare for women - the same arguments we had in the 1960s and 70s, and for decades before that time! It would be comical if it weren't so serious. It's a vicious circle, and women and their healthcare are caught in the middle.

Medical Misperceptions

Gynecologists treat women for a large portion of their lives, but generally speaking, they are not hormonal experts.

The public perception is that gynecologists are women's health experts. You would think by the nature of their specialty, they would have all the information on hormonal deficiencies and how to best treat them, wouldn't you? Sorry, no. They're surgeons and they like to deliver babies. They're not taught any more about hormones than a general practice physician. Seriously.

In reality, they'll often say "you're too young to have hormonal imbalances," or they'll tell you "there's no data to support hormone replacement therapy". However, there is plenty of data supporting hormone replacement therapy and its health benefits - most just haven't bothered to read it or learn it. It's baffling to me, especially since hormones play such a large part in a specialty based around fertility, reproductive health and family planning.

Lost Clinical Skills

Doctors in general are losing their clinical skills. We are commonly taught in medical school that 95 percent of a diagnosis will come from a patient's history, and yet somehow we have come to rely on labs instead of our own common sense and clinical know-how. We should be using labs to confirm our diagnosis, and not the other way around. So what did doctors do before labs? They examined a patient, asked a lot of questions and looked carefully through the person's chart and history. Today, patients often complain (and rightly so) that their doctor rushes through their exam and doesn't pay attention or listen to them.

Moreover, labs are not always accurate. For example, every day I see patients who are exercising and eating right, but they're still gaining weight, they feel cold all the time, they're fatigued, and losing their hair. These patients have all the telltale signs of hypothyroid, or low thyroid. Other doctors have told them their lab panel says their thyroid is normal, and more often than not, they are wrong.

Unfortunately, the most common lab test physicians order is the basic thyroid stimulating hormone (TSH) test, which often comes back in normal range – but that's only part of the picture. Doctors need to look for the sublevels - T3, T4, and reverse T3, which are more reliable and show the true colors of the thyroid function. (More on this later.)

If a patient walks into my office with these symptoms and their medical exam is consistent with thyroid issues — for instance, showing other signs of hypothyroidism such as slowed reflexes, slow heart rate and low temperature — I start them on treatment and then order the labs I described above. I haven't been wrong yet.

The Women's Health Initiative Media Frenzy

News reports on the Women's Health Initiative (WHI) – the biggest study ever done on synthetic hormone drugs – scared the hell out of women and doctors. Of course, it turns out the results of this complex study were skewed, misreported and misunderstood. Most prominently was the story featured on the cover of Newsweek on July 22, 2002, with the title, "Beyond Hormones: A New Study Raises Fears About the Risks For Millions Of Women. Here's What You Should Do."

Most women and even worse, most doctors, base their opinions and beliefs about hormone replacement therapy (HRT) on this study and the media hype surrounding it. What most don't realize is that this was a single, badly designed and highly flawed study on two bad synthetic drugs. First, the treatment group was older women who are misrepresentative of the population that usually uses HRT. James H. Clark, author of one of the papers critiquing the WHI study, wrote:

> "Most reproductive scientists believe that post-menopausal hormones should be used as preventive, not corrective therapy; therefore, treatment should begin during the menopausal transition."

The WHI study was based entirely on two synthetic drugs — Premarin and Prempro — that are not bio-identical (I'll talk more about this in a bit) and largely no longer used by medical professionals.

The media cherry picked statistically insignificant incidents and created false conclusions; shouting that women on HRT faced a 26 percent increase for risk of developing breast cancer. In reality, the number they chose to focus on was based on EIGHT more women having breast cancer in the Prempro portion of the study. Later analysis of the study actually showed no statistically significant increase for risk of breast cancer was found in the women in the Prempro study, and there was, in fact, a 23 percent

11

decrease in the Premarin group. Why wasn't the media shouting this from the rooftops? The widespread and irresponsible reporting of this single flawed study frightened women away from hormones therapies for the next decade. When it was discovered the study was mainly bunk, it got barely a blip on the media's radar. Even worse, because of this study, doctors became seriously concerned about liability — understandably, they didn't want to get sued if a woman got breast cancer. Many physicians still won't prescribe HRT, even if it's bio-identical, because their belief that HRT is harmful is rooted in the initial study and they haven't researched any further. However, I know the data. I've studied it inside and out for decades. There's far more good data and studies showing many types of HRT are safe and have positive effects on women's health. I've seen the same conclusions firsthand, reflected in the wonderful, positive results experienced by thousands of patients I've treated with bio-identical HRT.

Bio-identical Versus Synthetics

Pharmaceutical companies can't secure a patent on a molecule like testosterone or estradiol unless there's something unique about it, such as a special delivery system. Trying to patent molecules is like trying to patent a hamburger. The Vivelle-Dot, a bio-identical estrogen patch women wear on their skin, won a patent because it uses a unique delivery method. No company is going to invest millions or even billions of dollars to get a product FDA approved if they can't protect the patent.

The reality is that major pharmaceutical companies make ridiculous profits selling their brand name drugs for high cholesterol, stress, sleep disorders, migraines, and the like. Unfortunately they're allowed to advertise them directly to patients and market them to doctors (sometimes even providing incentives).

So it's Ambien for sleep problems. Imitrex for migraine headaches. Lipitor for high cholesterol. Xanax for anxiety. Lexapro or Prozac for depression. Of course, all of these drugs are highly profitable for the pharmaceutical companies that patented them. So here's your first health survival tip: All the symptoms these highly profitable drugs are designed to treat are most often related to hormonal deficiencies. Yes, hormonal deficiencies. Most health professionals are treating symptoms, and not the cause. Using HRT to effectively treat underlying hormone deficiencies in women can relieve symptoms, and eliminate the need for most or all of these medications in most patients. Now you understand why big pharma is fighting an all-out war against bio-identical hormones and other forms of HRT.

Money Talks

Big Pharma wants women to continue to take their brand name prescribed drugs for all the symptoms and conditions related to hormone deficiencies rather than going on hormone therapy, which can eliminate the need for many of their patented drugs, and they have the deep pockets to do it.

Lobbyists for the pharmaceutical industry are paid big bucks to try to kill access to non-patentable bio-identical hormones, and they continue to circulate bad information about HRT to do it.

Wyeth is working overtime trying to shut down compounding pharmacies, where most of the hormones we use are made, and insisting that doctors only be allowed to prescribe FDA-approved drugs (in other words, drugs developed, advertised, promoted and profited on by big pharma). If they succeed in their mission, it will be devastating for women.

Gender Bias

Men can get plenty of FDA-approved hormone products related to sexual dysfunction, but for years the FDA had yet to approve any testosterone products for women or any kind of drugs to help female sexual dysfunction. Unfair? You bet.

Finally, in 2015, the FDA approved a drug one; a horrible anti-depressant which causes such major side effects doctors need to become credentialed to prescribe it and women can't even drink alcohol while taking it! This is why women have sex in the first place, right??

Think about it: men can easily get erectile dysfunction medications, but women are finding it difficult to get the HRT they need to treat a variety of health conditions - and sexual dysfunction is just ONE of those conditions. The old double standard at work again?

When I was the Senior Medical Director at Procter and Gamble's pharmaceutical division, we tried to get a testosterone patch for women to market. The results of the WHI study on HRT had been reported about one year prior and everyone was worried that hormones, including testosterone, were killing women. The patch was approved for use in Europe and Australia in 2006, but the FDA blocked it here, citing concerns that testosterone replacement would cause increased risk of breast cancer and cardiovascular issues, even though the clinical trials for the patch never showed those results.

Ironically, testosterone has been used to treat women with breast cancer, and based on the data, actually lowers the risk of breast cancer in women. All studies done to date on low-dose testosterone replacement in women have showed no increase in cardiovascular risk or any other adverse effects of concern. The only proven side effects of properly dosed testosterone replacement therapy is an increased risk in facial hair — which menopausal women get anyway, and an increased risk for mild acne breakouts (these are usually temporary), which is why you need to go to a well-trained, well-educated doctor who knows what they are doing. Erectile dysfunction drugs can make a man go blind, deaf or even die, but there's no way the FDA will get between a man and his penis pills. But God forbid we get a little extra chin hair growth or a pimple!

So, here are the facts about testosterone replacement in women: if testosterone is given in too high of a dosage, it may cause excessive hair growth, acne, voice deepening, an enlarged clitoris, and cholesterol and liver abnormalities. All this fuss makes women worry they're going to turn into a hairy Sasquatch man, but that's not the case when the proper dosage is given. Once I tell women how much testosterone their bodies actually make to begin with, they're usually surprised.

However, estrogen can cause thickening of the uterine lining if it's not properly balanced by progesterone, which can lead to irregular bleeding and spotting. Estrogen itself will not cause breast cancer, but if a breast cancer cell is present and estrogen is prescribed, it will make it grow faster. Physicians must properly monitor women for side effects and understand the true risks.

Doctors & Patients Have Baggage

Many doctors think hormones are all about sex, and they are wrong. There are far more things at stake than simply getting your groove back in the bedroom. Hormone deficiencies have ramifications on cardiovascular health, weight gain, sugar metabolism, mood disorders and more. When hormones and sexual health come into play, many doctors complicate matters by bringing their own issues about women and sexuality into the mix. Due to their religious beliefs or ethnic background, they may believe women shouldn't have sex outside of wedlock. Others are simply uncomfortable or embarrassed talking to their patients about their sexuality.

Patients are often embarrassed to bring up sexual issues with their doctor, too. A study in the *Journal of the American Medical Association* found that while 85 percent of adults want to discuss sexual function with their doctors, 71 percent believe their doctor doesn't want to discuss it or doesn't have the time. Sixty-eight percent don't want to embarrass their doctor, and 76 percent thought no treatment was available for their problems. The study also reported "non-empathetic and/or judgmental responses, physician discomfort, concern about privacy and/or confidentiality, and lack of cultural sensitivity."

Bio-Identical HRT Versus Synthetic HRT

I have invested much of my time and energy researching, studying and understanding how hormones affect health in order to discover the truth about the pros and cons of HRT. I go out on a limb every day by treating hormone deficiencies in women and men through hormone therapy, but I know in my heart and educated mind that it is the right thing to do. The results speak for themselves.

I accept the risk of litigation because I know the data and understand the real risks, and I use compounded bio-identical hormones, and not synthetic. Bio-identical hormones are natural, plant-derived compounds with the same molecular structure as the hormones made by the human body. Unlike synthetic hormones, our bodies can readily recognize and metabolize them.

Since the 1930s, patients throughout Europe, Japan and the United States have successfully used bio-identical hormones. Study after study shows that when prescribed and administered correctly, bio-identical hormone pellets can help a variety of conditions, including depression, weight gain and osteoporosis. Pellets the size of a grain of rice are implanted under the skin of the buttocks. They don't present the potential hazards that synthetic hormones administered orally do, because they're not processed through the liver.

If they're so great, you might ask, why don't pharmaceutical companies market them? Since they're derived from plants, it's impossible for any drug manufacturer to get a patent. No patent, no big profit.

A trained pharmacist makes bio-identical hormones at a compounding pharmacy. Based on the prescription issued by a physician, the dosage is formulated and compounded to meet the specific needs for each patient – which is ideal, because as women know, one size does not fit all.

Bottom line: patients feel better and in many cases, we are able to get them off of multiple medications. I take calls daily from other physicians asking why I'm doing this, and have to defend my reasons. I've even created a 30-page document highlighting all the benefits and supporting data that I share with them. I battle the insurance companies, explaining health benefits that are derived from hormone replacement therapy; the long-term positive effects that can actually help keep patients healthier longer; and how in turn, these therapies can help lower healthcare costs by preventing chronic diseases from developing in the first place. Again, my goal as a doctor is to prevent disease, and BHRT is one of the best tools I have.

We're slowly making a difference, but we need more doctors and patients fighting the fight. Doctors need to keep up with medical journals and attend regular educational meetings about hormones and women's health. Medicine changes quickly, and you need a doctor who keeps up with it, instead of relying on what they originally learned in medical school for the next 40 or so years of their career.

I have witnessed firsthand all of the difficulties we face getting our voices heard, and I'm calling for a menopause revolution.

We're hot as hell, and we're not going to take it anymore!

CHAPTER THREE

EVERYTHING YOU EVER WANTED TO KNOW ABOUT HORMONES BUT DIDN'T KNOW HOW TO ASK: HORMONES 101

Let's get down and dirty about the business of what hormones are and what they do for us. It's OK if you want to skip ahead and come back to this chapter, but it's important to understand what each hormone does in the body, so you can understand what's going on in your body. Stick with me; I'll try to make it as painless as possible. We're going to go over testosterone, estrogen, progesterone and thyroid.

Strong Enough For a Man, But We Use It, Too

Testosterone is the hormone that makes guys "guys," giving them their rugged features, rippling muscles, sexy body and facial hair. Beyond that, how well do you really know it? Though it's strong enough for a man, women use it, too. It's also the hormone that makes women "women." As I mentioned previously, healthy women are meant to have about 60 percent estrogen and 40 percent testosterone in their body.

Testosterone helps keep up our energy, regulates our moods, and even helps us keep our feminine shape. OK, that last part usually comes as a surprise, but it's true: testosterone helps us burn sugar and keeps the weight off our middle (what you might know as the old "muffin top"). Testosterone also helps keep our breast tissue healthy and cancer- free.

In women, testosterone is made in the ovaries (90%) and

adrenal glands (10%). Testosterone is similar to estrogen in structure, however, it does very different, but complementary things for the body. Testosterone is actually quite nimble. Like estrogen, it can convert to other molecules. It can convert to estrogen as well as another hormone called 5-DHT. This is a more potent version of testosterone, which primarily shows its effects in the skin — for instance, it can cause acne and male pattern baldness. But 5-DHT cannot be converted into estrogen; it is too "manly."

So, what happens when your testosterone starts to decline? (Remember, this usually happens in our thirties). First, you start to notice less tolerance for stupid people and the stupid things people do. You lose your coping mechanism for life and sometimes, your filter. You start to become irritable and more moody. Some women become overtly depressed or anxious. I have seen patients develop severe anxiety, panic attacks and even the feeling of wanting to commit suicide. Mostly, though, women just don't feel anything anymore — they're apathetic. They wonder, "Is this is all life has to offer?" They say, "I have a wonderful life, I love my kids, I love my husband, I love my job, so why am I so unhappy?" Often, if they say this to doctors, they get prescribed antidepressants or, if they don't seek help, they may end up in divorce court.

I honestly believe that many couples break up when women start going through perimenopause and it's largely due to testosterone deficiency. These women feel different, and in turn their husbands may start to feel neglected. It's not the women's fault — it's simply the testosterone deficiency wreaking havoc on their moods and brain. Testosterone is Mother Nature's serotonin and affects how our brain processes information and how we feel. Most antidepressants increase serotonin levels so we can feel better. However, testosterone does this same thing and most women don't need antidepressants if they get testosterone replacement.

We almost certainly think of testosterone's role in the libido. Testosterone fires in the sexual centers in brain's limbic system (the innate, primal part of the brain) and promotes the desire for sex. Think Austin Powers: "Do I make you feel horny? Yeah, baby!" Without testosterone, we do not have or feel this "horniness," and this often leads to no desire at all. We love our partners, but just don't have it in us anymore to want sex.

That's why it's common for women to question, "I love my husband, but am I 'in love' with him?" and it can have devastating consequences. Women start to think it's a relationship problem, when it's really a hormone deficiency issue. However, over time, deficiencies and self- doubt can lead to relationship issues, because sex is the driver for emotional intimacy and physical connection between partners. It is what separates us from being "just friends."

Testosterone also makes our genitals (particularly the clitoris) spark with sensitivity and pleasure upon touch, hopefully leading to that almighty "O." It helps with intensity and longevity, and boosts our ability to climax more quickly. It provides the vestibule (the area surrounding the opening of the vagina) with lubrication, and enhances pleasure. It helps the uterus contract during orgasm, increasing intensity of the sensation. Without testosterone, everything takes longer and may be lackluster. Pair these physical responses with lack of desire, and it's really going to mess with our heads.

Our poor partners can't compete with a brain that feels nothing, and then when you finally do give in to sex, it simply doesn't feel as good as it once did. This opens the door for potential marital problems and affairs.

Testosterone is also essential for normal brain function, and in particular, executive function thinking. What's that? It helps us retain information, drives our short-term memory and recall, and the ability to process new abstract ideas. It gives us that "killer instinct" and the motivation essential to survival in a rapidly progressing work environment. Estrogen may help all the brain centers communicate with one another, but testosterone is specific to executive function. In other words, testosterone is the hunter and estrogen is the gatherer. When levels drop, it's no wonder our brains get foggy. Women think they are losing their minds and often become concerned that they're developing early Alzheimer's disease or dementia. Replacing testosterone helps maintain the brain's top performance.

For all the good, important tasks testosterone accomplishes, its most important role is to help us burn sugar. It helps prevent weight gain, as well as insulin resistance (a/k/a pre-diabetes). When we eat a meal, the food is digested, and converted into glucose to fuel our body. The speed of glucose conversion depends on the type of food we eat. For instance, if we eat a candy bar, our glucose levels spike very high immediately. This is challenging for the pancreas, as we end up using more insulin more rapidly, which in turn, causes very high and then very low blood sugar levels. These effects of these massive swings cause more harm to the body. As blood sugar drops, we start craving sugar, and the body begins to store more glucose as fat. Eventually, the ups and downs lead to pancreatic burnout. Now, we're entering weight gain territory, then it's on to pre-diabetes, and if left unchecked, we'll eventually arrive at diabetes.

So, how does testosterone affect sugar and pancreatic function? First, testosterone helps us move any immediate sugar in the bloodstream into the muscle, so the muscle can burn it cleanly. Second, testosterone helps us make more muscle cells so we can burn more sugar. This is why men lose weight faster than women. They have more muscle and more testosterone. Men are biologically set up to burn sugar easier than women. The truth hurts, doesn't it? I guess we have the all-important trump card — "Oh yeah, we can make babies and keep the human race going."

Many of my patients come in with pre-diabetic blood sugar levels, and within one month of treating them with testosterone, their sugar levels are normal. They were never truly pre-diabetic; it was simply a sign of testosterone deficiency. However, many providers don't realize this, and they start getting on our case to eat better and exercise (yeah, right — as if we weren't tired and busy enough). After we fail, they suggest you start medications like Metformin, which helps regulate blood sugars in prediabetics and diabetics.

If you're keeping track, the doctor now has us on antidepressants, anti-anxiety medications, diabetes medications and any number of supplements to help our memory and sex life. Better living through pharmaceuticals? It is depressing to know that so many of my colleagues are using medications as Band-Aids for symptoms of testosterone deficiency. These symptoms could be eliminated and good health restored if we simply gave women proper testosterone treatment for deficiencies.

When Mama Ain't Happy, Nobody's Happy

Estrogen is a pretty amazing substance. It's known as the "female" hormone, but it was present before humans ever came on the scene. Estrogen is found naturally in plants and. (If you've ever read about soy, you know this.) But did you know estrogen is present in sperm cells?

All men produce estrogen, just not as much as women do. On a day- to-day basis, men produce approximately 5 percent estrogen. All living species have estrogen in some degree or form.

Estrogen is one of the "heavy lifters" of the body and should not garner fear, but respect and admiration from patients and physicians. It's essential for everything in our bodies to run right. It feeds all of our cells and helps us maintain our vitality inside and out. When estrogens are balanced, the body fires on all four cylinders. When they're not, look out: "When mama ain't happy, no one's happy."

Estrogen's prime role in the body is for reproduction. We are born with eggs in our ovaries to propagate the gene pool. After puberty, every month the brain stimulates the ovaries to start maturing an egg for release and potential fertilization. It does this by increasing the level of estrogen in the bloodstream. Levels of estrogen must get high enough each month to allow for ovulation. If your ovaries don't make enough estrogen, you won't ovulate. This is why women's periods are very erratic when we're entering puberty and ovaries are new to the job, and again as we go through the phases of menopause. Initially, the ovaries are learning how to work, and at the end they just get tired, and our periods once again become erratic. When our period finally stops and the ovaries retire, we're in menopause. But estrogen doesn't just stimulate egg formation: It also helps the uterus prepare for the egg to implant by thickening the lining, and also improves genital health, allowing for comfortable and pleasurable intercourse.

However, when estrogen isn't helping the ovaries prepare for reproduction, it helps the body in many different ways:

- It helps prevent our bones from breaking down, keeping them strong, and works with testosterone to promote new bone growth.

- It stimulates collagen growth and helps keep cells hydrated, resulting in soft, supple, healthy skin.

- It facilitates proper communication between brain cells, keeping our mental function sharp.

- It protects us from heart disease by improving electrical conductivity, strengthening muscle cells, and increasing the heart wall function. It also keeps our blood vessels flexible by promoting endothelial wall dilation within the blood vessels.

These processes, along with hundreds of other day-to-day body functions all rely on proper estrogen levels. Without it, our bodies start to age rapidly and outwardly, we begin to show visible signs of aging. Our bodies begin to break down internally as well, putting us at higher risk for chronic illness.

Estrogen evokes fear in many, including too many medical professionals who should understand how it works in the body, but really don't. The key to understanding why bio-identical estrogens are safe is that not all estrogens are created equal. Cells in our bodies respond differently depending on the type of estrogen present and which cell receptors are on that cell taking in the estrogen. Think of a lock and a key. The estrogen is the key and the receptor is the lock. Some estrogens fit nicely into some locks, but not others. You need the right combination to open the lock in order to create the right positive effect for the body. Each woman has a different balance of keys and locks — none of us is exactly alike. That's why we shouldn't (and don't) prescribe the same doses of bio-identical hormones to every woman.

There are many different estrogens, but for simplicity's sake, we will talk about the big three: Estrone, estradiol, estriol.

Estrone (E1) – This is a moderate strength estrogen made in our fat cells. If we're overweight, an enzyme called aromatase converts estradiol to estrone in the fat cells. Estrone is weaker but more toxic, which is why more overweight women will have more

23

breast cancer. If you're overweight, you shouldn't take too much estradiol because it will convert to estrone.

Estradiol (E2) — This is the good, strong estrogen. It keeps us feeling great and keeps our body healthy. This is the one we want to replace. This is the estrogen contained in the Climara and Vivelle-Dot patches, troches and pellets we use in our practice.

Estriol (E3) – When pregnant, women make large amounts of estriol, and also in minute amounts when we're not pregnant. It's very weak and helps balance overall estrogen by blocking estrone's effects on estrogen- responsive cells, which is why some doctors and researchers think it protects the breasts. However, when this estrogen breaks down it makes a metabolite called 16-alpha hydroxyesterone that's toxic to breasts. Some providers don't prescribe it because of this conversion. Based on common sense biology, I believe that it is more likely to be protective because it's the hormone that protects both mother and baby during pregnancy. How it does this is not well understood.

In addition to having three different estrogens, women have different estrogen receptors that accept these estrogens differently. These are called ER alpha receptors and ER beta receptors. They're largely found in the breasts (Mother Nature's breast augmentation), heart, blood vessels, the uterine lining, brain cells, and bones. In fact, these receptors are found in almost every cell in the body.

ER alpha receptors are the "stimulator" receptors which cause growth in various systems in the body. ER beta receptors are the "dampening" receptors which are responsible for keeping ER alpha in check, by prompting cells to relax so they don't grow unregulated. When cells become unregulated, they can begin to rapidly multiply, resulting in uncontrolled rates of growth. Ultimately, these cells have the potential to mutate and become cancerous.

For example, the breasts and uterus contain both receptors, but ER beta receptors are most predominant. ER alpha receptors take in estrogen, causing the breast tissue and uterine lining to grow during certain times in our cycle, as well as reproductive lives. As we learned earlier, the ER beta receptors fend off the ER alpha so that the cells don't grow out of control. The more ER beta

24

signaling there is in the breast and uterine lining, the fewer incidences of breast and uterine cancer.

So the ER beta protects lung tissue, the ovaries, the colon, the immune system, the bladder, the brain and serotonin neurotransmission, and every other cell in the body, just like ER alpha receptors. We need both receptors to live happy and healthy lives. However, the ER beta receptors are the ones specifically responsible for helping to prevent cancers in women.

Increase ER Beta and Decrease ER Alpha

So how do we increase our ER beta and decrease our ER alpha? ER beta is increased by eating certain foods; as well as vitamins D and E, and maintained through healthy levels of estriol and testosterone. Foods containing plant isoflavones (soy), whole grains, cruciferous vegetables (like cabbage, brussel sprouts, broccoli and kale) help promote ER beta dominance, but also help decrease inflammation in the body. Estriol and testosterone increase ER beta dominance and decrease the ER alpha signaling, helping to reduce cancers overall, and in particular, breast cancer. On the flip side, diets low in phytoestrogens and cruciferous vegetables, when coupled with low estriol and low testosterone levels increase the risk of ER alpha signaling and cancers.

ER alpha signaling is increased by: being overweight, eating a diet that's high in junk foods, increased levels of stress, exposure to synthetic estrogens, excessive alcohol consumption, low functioning thyroid (another reason to replace thyroid), vitamin D deficiency and bad genetics.

If you consider the three estrogens previously mentioned: Estrone binds more strongly to the ER alpha receptors, causing more cell growth and increasing the risk of cancer. Estriol binds more predominantly to ER beta receptors, decreasing cell growth and the risk of cancer. Estradiol is well balanced between ER alpha and ER beta. This balance makes it the ideal estrogen for promoting good cell growth in tissues, but it knows when it needs to take a breather.

Given this information, it makes sense that women with estrogen deficiencies need the good, well-balanced estrogen that helps promote healthy, stable growth in tissue, while simultaneously keeping cell growth in check. This is why I prescribe estradiol for women — the bio- identical "good," strong estrogen.

Many pharmaceutical companies are trying to make "designer" estrogens that positively affect the ER alpha receptors, while using ER beta control on the bad effects of overstimulation. Medications such as Tamoxifen help protect the breast, but still have the negative alpha effect on the uterus, increasing the risk for developing uterine cancer. Raloxifene provides the positive stimulatory effect on ER alpha on the bone, and a positive ER beta effect on the breast and uterus. Like Tamoxifen, Raloxifene provides breast protection, but unlike Tamoxifen, it does not increase the risk for uterine cancer. Once you understand the types of estrogens and estrogen receptors, you better understand the benefits of these drugs, as well as their potential side effects.

Progesterone - Estrogen's Ugly Stepsister

Progesterone is related to estrogen, and estrogen needs progesterone in order to properly maintain our reproductive capability. But unlike estrogen (the "feel good" hormone), progesterone typically doesn't make us feel good – it's more like the sister who constantly nags you. High progesterone levels are thought to be partly responsible for symptoms of premenstrual syndrome (PMS), such as breast tenderness, bloating and mood swings.

You're probably thinking, "Then what good is progesterone? Why do we need her, if all she does is cause us grief?"

Progesterone can be annoying, but like the nagging sibling, you really need her in your life, you just have to find the balance. When she's not around, you start to notice. Your periods stop coming regularly, and you'll be left wondering what's happening to your body. Without progesterone, all of your hormones will be out of balance, and you won't feel well.

Let's go over the details of what progesterone does and how it acts in the body. It has many functions, but its biggest and most important job is to prepare the body for pregnancy. During our reproductive years, the pituitary gland in the brain generates hormones: follicle-stimulating hormone (FSH) and luteinizing hormone (LH). These cause a new egg to mature and be released from its ovarian follicle each month. As the follicle develops, it produces estrogen, which thickens the lining of the uterus. Progesterone levels rise in the second half of the menstrual cycle, and following the release of the egg (ovulation), the ovarian tissue that replaces the follicle continues to produce progesterone.

So, to review, estrogen stimulates growth of the uterine lining, causing it to thicken before you ovulate each month. Progesterone gears up in the second half of the menstrual cycle, getting everything prepared for pregnancy; causing the endometrium to secrete special proteins, preparing it to receive and nourish an implanted fertilized egg. If the egg doesn't implant, estrogen and progesterone levels drop, the endometrium breaks down, and we have our period.

If a pregnancy occurs, progesterone is produced in the placenta, and levels remain elevated throughout the pregnancy. The combination of high estrogen and progesterone levels suppress further ovulation during pregnancy. Progesterone also primes the breast to be able to deliver milk for breastfeeding.

In order to ovulate, you need adequately high estrogen levels during mid-cycle. If you don't ovulate, you won't produce progesterone. You might say, "Hey, that doesn't sound so bad. If I don't get enough progesterone, I won't have PMS, right?" Wrong. Everything has to work in concert. If your estrogen is chronically low, especially to the point where you're not having periods, it also can make you weepy, bloated and cause breast tenderness - similar to PMS.

The idea is to keep everything in balance. Think of the three hormones as siblings. Testosterone is the happy-go-lucky brother who keeps the peace between estrogen (the beautiful, popular sister everyone loves) and progesterone (the ugly stepsister). When they're all together and doing their chores like they're supposed to, the body is happy. Unfortunately, during perimenopause, testosterone is always the first to move out of the house, so the brother who would normally keep the sisters in line is nowhere to be found. That makes the symptoms from the fluctuating estrogen and progesterone levels even worse. And that, my friends, is why perimenopause sucks.

Thyroid Hormones: Keep your Motor Running

The thyroid, as mentioned in Chapter 1, is the engine of our body. When the engine slows down or speeds up too much, you won't feel good. We need the engine to run not too fast, and not too slow, but just right.

To recap, the signs of low thyroid (a slow engine) include fatigue, weight gain, intolerance to cold, hair loss, muscle aches, constipation, irritability, depression and memory loss.

High thyroid (a fast engine), often called overactive thyroid (hyperthyroid), can also cause fatigue, along with diarrhea, intolerance to heat, sweatiness, nervousness, anxiety, high blood pressure, itching, rapid or irregular pulse, difficulty sleeping and weight loss. Although I know many women who would love to have a race car engine because it speeds up metabolism, it's just as damaging to the body as low thyroid.

Low functioning thyroid, or hypothyroidism, is much more common than hyperthyroid. Estimates range, but approximately 1 in 3 women and 1 in 5 men will have a low functioning thyroid (hypothyroidism) by the time they hit 50. Many women I meet are hypothyroid and have no idea, because they've been tested and told their thyroid is functioning fine.

So what makes these hormones that control so much of how we feel? It's the thyroid gland, a bow tie-shaped gland in the front of our neck. If it gets swollen, we call it a goiter. This can happen with both low and high thyroid, but it's most commonly found with low thyroid. It's easily treatable and not serious in most cases. Once you get the proper thyroid medication, it's resolved.

The brain is the thyroid's boss. The thyroid's job is to secrete a molecule (or pro-hormone) called T4. When it's making enough T4, the brain sends the thyroid a signal that says "Yep, everything is A-OK up here," so it keeps producing the same level of T4. If it's not making enough, the brain sends out TSH, or thyroid stimulating hormone that says "Hey, lazy! Ramp up the production!" and in response, the thyroid begins pumping out more T4. Unfortunately, this is only half the story, but it's usually the only half doctors check, which is why the hypothyroid diagnosis is so often missed.

Many women make enough T4, but the problem is that T4 is an inactive molecule that needs to convert to its active T3 form. T3 is the molecule that triggers a response in the body's cells. Every cell in the human body has receptors that accept the T3 molecule. If the T4 does not properly convert to T3, the thyroid can make all the T4 it wants, but it will never trigger the appropriate cellular responses. They simply won't fire properly.

To make matters worse, there's a little decoy molecule called reverse T3, which can sit in the thyroid receptors on the cells, blocking the active T3 molecule from docking and talking to the cell. If you block T3 from getting into the cell's receptors, the cells never activate. This means you can have normal thyroid function, but since the T3 cannot enter the cells, you are 'functionally hypothyroid' on a cellular level.

To recap, there are three ways the system can go awry:

1. **You don't make enough T4.** This is easy to spot, because doctors commonly test for T4 levels, and the brain hormone TSH (thyroid stimulating hormone) will show up as high. If the thyroid is not doing its job, the brain uses TSH to whip the thyroid into manufacturing more T4. The lazier the thyroid is, the more it gets beaten into producing more. (Picture the TSH as a mean boss with a whip, and the slower the worker, the more he gets whipped.) Since most doctors only check for TSH and T4 levels, if they don't see anything wrong, they say the thyroid is fine. But they're missing the most essential parts of the picture.

2. **The inactive T4 does not convert well to the active T3.** The enzyme 5-deiodinase is necessary to convert T4 into active T3. Without enough of this enzyme, your body won't be able to "kick" the extra iodine molecule off the T4 to convert into the active T3. Too much iodine in the diet or in supplements can inhibit this process.

3. **The active T3 can't get into the receptors.** If a doctor doesn't check T3 and reverse T3 levels, they cannot get the true picture of a patient's thyroid health. Many of my new patients present with a full set of symptoms consistent with low thyroid, and the clinical exam that supports this, but

their T4 and TSH levels are normal. However, if I look at T3 and reverse T3 levels, I can easily see the problem. Most often, the body isn't converting T4 to active T3. But some women have too much reverse T3 blocking the receptors. This can be caused by medications, adrenal dysfunction, stress and other factors. Some women have just one of these thyroid problems, but many have all three issues.

A less common disorder is too much thyroid, or hyperthyroidism. This is the exact opposite of hypothyroidism. The thyroid makes too much T4, and the whole body is hyper-activated. Lab tests will show too much T4, too much T3 and a very low TSH. (The TSH doesn't need to whip the worker, because he's already working fast and hard, so labs will show decreased levels.)

As you can see, unless all of the levels are tested, you can't properly diagnose thyroid disorders, and hypothyroidism is the one most often missed. Luckily, hypothyroidism is usually not difficult to treat. It requires taking a pill each day. However, an incomplete diagnosis will affect proper treatment of the disorder. For instance, a doctor might give a patient medication solely to increase T4. But it won't matter if you're not successfully converting T4 to T3, or if you have a lot of reverse T3 blocking the effects of T3. You can give someone all of the T4 in the world, but the patient will never improve. You need to administer T3.

From the early 1900s, a common thyroid pill made by Armour (from crushed-up pig thyroid) containing T4 and T3 was used to treat hypothyroid. The first ever thyroid medication, it was effective and widely prescribed. Today, the most popular medication used to treat thyroid in conventional practices, including endocrinologists, is a synthetic hormone called Synthroid. Made by a large pharmaceutical company, it's the top-selling thyroid medication in the U.S., and one of the top-selling drugs in America. The problem is that Synthroid only contains T4. So if you're hypothyroid and on Synthroid and you still feel like crap, it's not your imagination, it's a matter of simple chemistry.

If you have a T4 disorder, Synthroid is fine, but if you don't covert T4 well to T3 or you have a lot of reverse T3, you need to take an additional medication called Cytomel (which is pure T3) or better yet, use a drug like Armour, which contains both T3 and T4.

So why is this less-effective medication so popular now? After Synthroid was launched, the company began an extensive marketing and rewards campaign inside the medical community, using authoritative figures to create brand loyalty. Gradually, many endocrine societies and even endocrinologist experts began stating that Armour should not be used. Today, medical students are taught in schools not to prescribe it. But it's all hogwash, pardon the pun, because Armour is safe, effective and cheap; and most of my patients don't mind that it's made from pigs. I do have some patients who are highly allergic to certain substances and can't take pig thyroid, and some Jewish patients who don't wish to take it because of religious observance. But roughly 90 percent of my patients are on Armour and they do very well.

Big Pharma has a vested interest in making Synthroid the go-to drug for low thyroid, even when it doesn't effectively address the patients' problem. If you take Synthroid and don't feel better and your doctor refuses to prescribe anything else, see another doctor.

One size does not fit all in medicine, and when it comes to hormones — including thyroid — this definitely holds true.

CHAPTER FOUR

PSYCHO BITCH SYNDROME: TESTOSTERONE DEFICIENCY IN THE 20S

Testosterone deficiency can occur as early as a woman's twenties, and it's more common than you'd think. Even though most women don't start perimenopause until their forties, roughly 20 percent of younger women will already have a testosterone deficiency in their twenties due to their genetic makeup, environmental exposures such as alcohol and drug use, pesticides, radiation exposure, etc. Even more women - perhaps a third of ALL women in their twenties - will have testosterone deficiencies because so many doctors unknowingly prescribe medications that reduce testosterone levels, and worse yet, they don't recognize the effects. The most common offender is oral contraceptives. Oral contraceptive pills are widely prescribed and used by millions of women for a variety of reasons besides contraception, often for years at a time without a break.

There's no doubt that "The Pill" launched a new era of freedom for millions of women, allowing them an effective way to take control of their family planning and prevent pregnancy. The Pill is widely credited for sparking the Sexual Revolution of the 1960s. However, there were unintended consequences far beyond the religious and ethical debates that continue to this day. The reality is that oral contraceptives rob the body of testosterone, but nobody bothered to explain this to women; let alone what the loss of this key hormone might actually do to their bodies. Perhaps it's buried somewhere in the miles of fine print in the massive packet inserts that are routinely tossed out each month. (I'll save you the trouble of looking: it's not.)

32

In order to understand this important point, you first have to understand how oral contraceptives work in the body. Oral contraceptives shut down the ovaries to prevent ovulation. No egg to meet up with sperm, no issue. Here's the problem: ovaries are not just about eggs. Their primary function is to manufacture hormones the body needs, so shutting down the hormone factory can hatch a bundle of unexpected problems.

Most oral contraceptives are a combination of synthetic estrogen and progesterone that replace what our ovaries would normally produce. Here's the key: what they don't replace is testosterone, and our ovaries manufacture most of it. In fact, it's 40% of our hormonal makeup, so already things have the potential to get ugly; and of course, it comes with a bonus gift.

Oral contraceptives process through the liver, producing a protein that starts to bind up the remaining testosterone made by the adrenal glands, and another that binds the "free thyroid" hormone needed to fuel metabolism. (We'll review this in more depth later.) We've already seen that testosterone deficiency, or low T, causes weight gain and fatigue, lowers libido and increases insulin resistance; raising our risk for developing diabetes, heart disease, strokes, and other serious conditions.

The widely used "low estrogen" pills are worst of all as they contain lots of progesterone, the PMS hormone that makes us gain weight, bloat, and feel irritable before we start our periods. High progesterone, along with low T and little to no estrogen, are going to cause us more problems; so these types of pills should only be used to control heavy bleeding or in women with PCOS. Even then, they're not ideal.

Oral Contraceptives: The Hidden Side Effects

Let's look at the case of Ashley, 27. Like many women her age, Ashley started taking birth control pills for contraception and to regulate her periods. Ashley is sexually active with her boyfriend, Zach, but more importantly, she has heavy, unpredictable periods that interfere with her ability to enjoy a basic quality of life.

Before she started taking the Pill, Ashley menstruated heavily and suddenly at unexpected intervals. She could have a period for three days, and three weeks later, start again and bleed for 10 days.

Then it could be five or six weeks before she had another one. She never knew. When she was in high school, it wasn't uncommon for her to soak through her jeans while sitting in class. She'd have to call her mom to pick her up so she could go home and change. Going to the beach or a public pool caused serious anxiety, so she'd put in a tampon every time. The Pill makes her periods run like clockwork, so she's never unpleasantly surprised.

However, there's a trade-off. Over the course of about a year, being on oral birth control pills caused Ashley's testosterone levels to plummet. Until now, she was a hot number who enjoyed running and working out at the gym, but she began experiencing fatigue, lack of muscle endurance, and more aches and pains than usual. She also gained 10 pounds rapidly due to sugar cravings, and because she's too tired to go to the gym, it's tough to keep the weight off. Lack of exercise also does nothing to temper her mood swings, anxiety, terrible PMS and debilitating migraines. Worst of all, she's lost interest in sex, experiences difficulty reaching climax, and even has pain during intercourse. Zach, who's starting to think she's "psycho," is considering going out with other women.

Ashley is questioning her sanity, too. She can't understand why all of these changes are happening to her and knows there's something off, so she turns to her trusty pal, the Internet. After Googling some women's health sites, she reads about hormonal problems and changes. Most of what she reads is directed towards women at the onset of menopause, or perimenopause, but she can't help but notice her symptoms mirror everything she's reading about.

Ashley thinks, "Hey, that's me," so she sees her gynecologist and tells him about her symptoms and the online research she's done. By the way, doctors just *love it* when patients self-diagnose using the Internet. Right off the bat, he's defensive and irritated with her. He tells her she's too young to have hormone deficiency, and advises her to get more rest, reduce her stress and consider using massage and erotic videos to help her get in the mood. If a doctor ever tells you this, by the way, walk — no, RUN out of the office immediately! It's condescending and rude, and also tells you they know absolutely nothing about female sexuality.

Ashley protests, so her doctor relents and tells her she can try a different birth control pill. He goes into his sample closet and grabs a pack of pills he recently got from his pharmaceutical rep, all without diagnosing what Ashley really needs. She takes the pack of new pills, and doesn't feel any improvement at all. And it's back to square one.

What's Really Happening to Ashley

As I described earlier, most methods of hormonal birth control are designed to stop the ovaries from ovulating, or releasing an egg each month. In essence, they stop working. That's good, because it prevents pregnancy and gives women control over family planning. But remember, the ovaries make the estrogen, testosterone and progesterone the body needs to function properly.

Once again, the unintended consequences of using most hormonal birth control methods (whether oral or non-oral, except for Mirena® IUD) is that they STOP your ovaries from making hormones that your body desperately needs. Oral birth control pills give back estrogen (although often not enough) and progesterone, but do not replace the missing testosterone.

To review: when the ovaries are working unsuppressed by the birth control pills, they produce 90 percent of the body's daily requirement of testosterone. The adrenal glands produce roughly 10 percent. If you use a non-oral hormonal birth control method like NuvaRing®, Ortho Evra® patch or Mirena® IUD, you at least get to keep that 10 percent from the adrenal glands. If you use the Pill, you lose all of it. So how does this happen?

When pills are taken by mouth, they go through the stomach, intestines and finally the liver. The liver metabolizes the hormones in the contraceptive pill to make them available to the body via the blood stream. During this process, the liver kicks out clotting factors that increase the risk of developing blood clots as well as a hormone called SHBG (serum hormone binding globulin). This big protein molecule loves to bind up other hormones and testosterone is its favorite victim. Now the testosterone that is biologically active (free T) is bound and unavailable. It's completely depleted.

It's this deficiency that's causing Ashley's symptoms — the aches, pains, migraines, sugar cravings and pain during sex. So the Pill can be good and evil: while it can regulate periods, decreases acne, lessen cramping, and most importantly, prevent pregnancy, it also can have nefarious short and long term effects.

At a conference in August 2012, I attended a seminar by Dr. Andrew Goldstein, president of the International Society for the Study of Women's Sexual Health. He said oral birth control pills are the number one cause of pelvic pain during intercourse. The opening of the vagina, called the vulvar vestibule, requires adequate estrogen and testosterone levels to remain healthy and pain-free during sex. Oral birth control alters these levels. One study suggests women who use hormonal contraception are more than six times more likely to develop pelvic pain syndromes. Stopping the pills may not resolve the symptoms. It might actually require estrogen and testosterone cream applied directly to the area to heal the tissues.

That's vitally important information women need to know when considering birth control methods. So what's the answer?

First, we need a primer on exactly how our cycles and hormones work. During the first half of a woman's menstrual cycle, estrogen rises, which helps thicken the uterine lining. Estrogen is the "feel good" hormone — we feel our best during this stage. Estrogen levels must get to a certain point to make an egg pop out of the ovary, and when it finally does, look out.

The egg comes out usually midway during our cycle, around day 14, and starts to produce progesterone. Now we're in the second half of the cycle, and this is when we don't feel so wonderful. Progesterone's job is to prepare the body for pregnancy in case the egg implants. It makes the uterine lining fluffy and soft, like a feather bed. It's preparing for a baby to nestle in there for the next nine months. Progesterone wants us to slow down, so it stimulates GABA receptors in our brain and makes us tired. We are woman; hear us snore!

Progesterone also wants the baby to get plenty of nutrition, so it makes us crave sugar. Also, it makes us retain water to help hydrate the baby. And then it makes our breasts swell in order to prepare us to breastfeed. All this is great for making babies, but not so hot for just about everything else, and it's hard not to let it show. And this, ladies, is what we know all too well as PMS. Men just call it "Oh, hell, it's that time of the month again," and recommend running for cover.

The egg will live 14 days, and if it's not fertilized, it dies. Once the egg dies, (usually the day before our period starts) our progesterone levels plummet, destabilizing the uterus and prompting bleeding — that fluffy "feather" bed meant for the would-be baby is no longer needed, so out it goes.

Estrogen levels are also at their lowest point the day the period starts, so the brain starts pumping out a follicle stimulating hormone (FSH). FSH whips the ovary into making estrogen, so the levels slowly rise, and the cycle starts over again. Once we get past the initial cramping, around day three to five of our period, we start to feel better. As estrogen rises, we're no longer crabby, tired, bloated, sugar-seeking missiles – hooray, we are feeling normal again!

Now back to birth control pills. The pills are a combination of estrogen and progesterone in some ratio. Many doctors and patients have been taught to believe a low-estrogen pill is better. But the lower the estrogen, the higher the progesterone – OMG, it's attack of the PMS hormone! We are basically tricking our bodies into PMS mode all the time, while creating estrogen deficiency symptoms like hot flashes, night sweats and more. So you get all this PLUS the newly hatched testosterone deficiency. Sounds fun, yes?

However, every woman is different, and not all birth control pills are created equal. Low-estrogen pills can have benefits for some women, like those with heavy bleeding. If you are at risk for breast cancer or for clots that can cause heart attacks and stroke — especially if you're over 35 and a smoker — then you should not take oral birth control pills at all. You can use contraceptives like the Mirena® IUD® or NuvaRing® that aren't processed through the liver, which does not increase the clotting risk.

For most of us, more estrogen is better. Estrogen is the "feel good" hormone, remember? And progesterone, especially the synthetic version, is more dangerous overall than estrogen was ever accused of being. This is all common sense if you know and understand the menstrual cycle. When doctors help women consider their birth control choices, they have to know what they're treating. Unfortunately, most women take the same brand of pills for years, not realizing that number one, they don't have to feel cruddy all the time, and number two, these pills are slowly killing them, and I mean this *literally*. How?

Maintaining high progesterone levels over a long period of time leads to a condition called metabolic syndrome. Women start to gain weight, especially in the midsection where it's most dangerous. They show abnormalities in their cholesterol panel. They start to show sugar problems that can lead to pre-diabetes, and that can lead to diabetes. Over three short years, women will develop a high risk for heart attack and stroke.

Back to Ashley. She remains frustrated. She feels like the doctor rush through the visit, patting her on her head and telling her she's in perfect health, and has nothing to worry about. This makes her doubt her sanity even more. After all, doctors know more than patients, right? Yes and no. Many doctors bring in their own personal biases and education levels. It doesn't mean doctors are bad or want to hurt women's health, more often than not, it's an unintended consequence of their lack of knowledge and training. Like 75 to 80 percent of doctors, Ashley's doctor just doesn't get it. These uninformed doctors can't believe a young woman in her twenties or thirties could possibly have hormonal problems. Since she doesn't outwardly show any serious signs of illness, he just wants to move Ashley through the office within the allotted 10 minutes and not get bogged down.

Despondent and confused, Ashley poured out her heart to her mother, who sees me for her own hormone issues. Bingo! Ashley makes an appointment. Right away, I recommend that she switch to a non-oral birth control method. Mirena® IUDs, NuvaRing®, Ortho Evra® patches (The Patch) — any of these methods will work better at maintaining that last 10 percent of the body's natural testosterone that comes from the adrenal glands, which can be enough for younger women without giving additional systemic testosterone replacement. Over time, they may still eventually develop testosterone deficiency as that 10 percent is no longer able to meet their body's physiological needs, but it could take years.

As mentioned earlier, stopping birth control pills doesn't always restore healthy tissue in the vaginal opening. In Ashley's case, I prescribe a compounded estrogen and testosterone cream to be applied to the opening of her vagina to help restore normal, healthy tissue and decrease the pain associated with sex.

If a woman wants to continue to use birth control pills (for example, she likes the convenience, or she's squeamish about inserting a NuvaRing® into the vagina, fearful of IUDs, or has trouble wearing The Patch because she swims or sweats heavily), it's OK; we just need to replace testosterone. However, it's best to avoid testosterone replacement in younger women who want to get pregnant or who aren't being completely careful about using contraception. When a woman's on testosterone replacement, there's a higher risk of having a female baby with ambiguous genitalia or conversion to male genitals. It's rare, but it's a real risk. But don't panic!

The good news is that women with a severe testosterone deficiency can go on testosterone replacement, and come off of it when they want to start a family. Unlike estrogen, testosterone doesn't get stored inside your fat cells, so you can stop it at any time — it takes a subcutaneous pellet about four to five months to totally deplete. Or you can use gels or creams, which leave the body within three to five days. But the best course, if you're unsure when you want to conceive, is to not use testosterone replacement therapy at all.

Ashley isn't married yet, but she thinks if it "just happened," Zach would be ready to a daddy. As I mentioned earlier, I recommended using an alternate form of birth control. Ashley chooses the NuvaRing® and finds it's much more convenient than the Pill — she simply inserts it, and doesn't have to think about it for the next three weeks.

It works. Ashley feels better physically and has started working out again. She eats better and has dropped those annoying 10 pounds, which has improved her mood as well. Her PMS is no longer at "psycho" levels, and her sex drive has returned, much to Zach's delight. After two or three months of using the prescribed compounded estrogen and testosterone cream, the pain she felt at the vaginal opening during sex went away.

Polycystic Ovarian Syndrome (PCOS)

The exception to the rule for testosterone and the positive effects it can have is when a woman has Polycystic Ovarian Syndrome (PCOS). This is a condition in which a woman has an imbalance of female sex hormones. It may lead to menstrual cycle changes, cysts in the ovaries, trouble getting pregnant and other health issues. These women have an altered balance of estrogen, progesterone and androgens (testosterone) levels in the body, with higher levels of androgens than are normal.

We don't completely understand why or how the changes in their hormone levels occur. The changes make it harder for a woman's ovaries to release fully grown (mature) eggs. Normally, one or more eggs are released during a woman's cycle (Ovulation). In PCOS, mature eggs are not released from the ovaries. Instead, they can form very small cysts in the ovary, and eventually these changes can contribute to infertility, and the cysts can become enlarged, more painful and sometimes even burst.

The other symptoms of this disorder are also due to hormone imbalances. These include: irregular periods or no period, increase in facial hair or overall body hair, increase in acne, deeper voice, enlarged clitoris, and decreased breast size. These women also have an ongoing struggle with weight gain and have an increased risk of developing pre- diabetes or diabetes.

Most of the time, PCOS is diagnosed in the 20s or 30s. However, it may also effect teenage girls. The symptoms often begin when a girl's periods start. Women with this disorder often have a mother or sister who has symptoms similar to those of PCOS. These women should not be given testosterone, as it will make things worse. The goal of treatment in this patient population is to stop the ovary from functioning (lowering the androgens) and control the sugar abnormalities that largely contribute to the infertility, weight gain and cardiovascular risk.

Happily, PCOS is not common, occurring in perhaps 5 to 20 percent of women, depending on the study consulted. For most of us, testosterone is a wonderful substance that keeps us balanced and healthy, so we need to make sure we have an ideal amount.

Now that you understand how oral contraceptives work, here's the bottom line: it's your body, so remember you need to maintain a good balance of estrogen and progesterone. Know how to recognize the signs and symptoms of testosterone deficiency, which can safely be replaced before things get out of control and create bigger problems.

CHAPTER FIVE

YOU'VE LOST THAT LOVIN' FEELING: TESTOSTERONE DEFICIENCY AND SEXUAL RESPONSE CHANGES IN THE 30S

In the classic film Annie Hall, Woody Allen's character Alvy Singer, and Diane Keaton's character Annie Hall are seeing their therapists at the same time, which is shown on a split screen.

Alvy Singer's Therapist: How often do you sleep together?

Annie Hall's Therapist: Do you have sex often?

Alvy Singer: [lamenting] Hardly ever. Maybe three times a week.

Annie Hall: [annoyed] Constantly. I'd say three times a week.

It's no surprise to anyone who's in, or has ever been in a relationship that emotional and sexual responses differ between men and women. Understanding these differences will go a long way towards creating happier couples. Hormone health often plays a role, too, as we'll see in the case of Melissa, 32, and her husband Eduardo.

These two are suffering from the "second year slump," which happens in nearly every relationship. The first year, their marriage was full of fireworks. It was all they could do to not paw at each other under the table at a restaurant. They made out like horny teenagers in the car before going home.

Sometime during the second year, Melissa started to fizzle out. Physically, she feels fine and doesn't have any symptoms of depression or anxiety. She simply doesn't initiate sex like she used to, and Eduardo feels like she may not be attracted to him anymore. He feels cheated and unhappy with the changes in their sex life, and now the marriage is in trouble. Her constant rotten moods have also caused him to pull away, and he's starting to go to lunch a lot more often with a woman at the office and confide in her about his unhappiness.

It's a vicious circle: Melissa doesn't have "that loving feeling" all the time anymore, which makes Eduardo grouchy, which in turn makes Melissa feel worse, which does nothing to make her want him more often. On top of all of this, when Melissa and Eduardo do have sex, they fall prey to many of the media images of sex and what's "normal" for couples.

Men tend to turn on like a light bulb but women turn on like an oven. It takes more time for us to heat up. But pornography and mainstream movies tend to show women dramatically flailing around having high- decibel orgasms, all within a few seconds of intercourse; which is completely unrealistic and can make both parties feel like losers if the woman takes more than a few minutes to orgasm. Melissa often gets anxious if she doesn't meet these ridiculous time frames, which makes it even more difficult for her to climax. Another vicious circle!

In addition, all of the wildly creative positions filmmakers like to show on screen are based in fiction and fantasy, not reality. It's impossible for women to orgasm in more than a few positions because 1. There must be enough clitoral stimulation, 2. Most women need some kind of tension or pressure in their thighs to drive tension in the pelvis or uterus, and 3. More time is often required — men can orgasm rather quickly (oh, don't some of us know THAT all too well!) while the average time for women is usually 15 to 20 minutes without the aid of a vibrator. Women, if you need to show your partner where your clitoris exactly is and what it needs, don't be shy! I promise you'll both be happier in the long run.

After mustering all of her confidence and overcoming her reluctance, Melissa confides to her doctor that something feels wrong. She doesn't understand why she doesn't get that sexual rush from Eduardo anymore. She's sure she still loves him, and is starting to think the problem is with her. Is there anything the doctor can do?

Uh-oh. Melissa's doctor, like most, is unprepared for this situation. She's perfectly knowledgeable and trained in everything from allergies to heart disease, but she's uncomfortable talking about sex with her patients. She doesn't understand what's going on physically, so she suggests Melissa and Eduardo see a "couples counselor" for therapy. They go on a retreat, and agree to schedule regular "date nights" that will always end with sex. Eduardo is OK with this, because he knows he will at least be getting some action on a regular basis.

Therapy and mandatory date nights aren't making Melissa feel any better, so she goes back to the doctor, who misdiagnoses Melissa's lack of sex drive as depression. She prescribes an antidepressant. Double uh- oh. What this doctor, like most, doesn't understand is that Melissa's feelings are totally normal and predictable, and by prescribing an antidepressant, she's screwed with Melissa's hormones, amplifying her problems. The second most common cause of low libido for women in their 20s and 30s is antidepressants. Most of these medications will sap your sex drive faster than your husband can say, "My mom's coming to visit for a month."

What most doctors aren't taught in medical school (or beyond) is that Melissa's sexual feelings for her husband are completely normal for this stage of their relationship. They've simply evolved due to natural biological and emotional changes. It's called entering a "sexually neutral state." Wait - that doesn't sound good, does it? Realize that the term "sexually neutral state" doesn't mean women don't want sex; it simply means *they just need a bit more time and attention to feel like having sex.*

Generally, once past the "jumping each other's bones" phase, men still need sex to relax, and women need to relax to have/ enjoy sex. Sorry to burst that romantic bubble, but this happens to virtually all women. Don't freak out, though. It's all about understanding what's happening and working through it all to benefit the relationship. If you don't even know what's happening, it's hard to recognize how to remedy it. Knowledge is power. So let's dig in.

Research into human sexual response began back in the late 1950s with pioneers William Masters and Virginia Johnson.

Masters & Johnson's theory was that male and female sexual response is linear, with minor exceptions. Men go through the stages of excitement, reach the plateau stage (the part where they think about baseball so they don't orgasm too soon), which is followed by orgasm and refractory or recovery stage. Women go through the same linear model, but there are three variations on their theme.

Masters and Johnson decided women could 1. Respond the same as men, 2. Go through excitement, plateau, and then go down to resolution with no orgasm, or 3. Go from excitement to orgasm in a rapid uptick and back down. However, in the late 1990s and early 2000s, a new intimacy-based model came about that better explains a lot of differences between men and women, and there's much more going on than meets the eye.

Most women in a new relationship will experience a similar level of sexual desire or hunger as a man. They feel the same kind of "rush" of sexual arousal and desire, which usually leads to sexual intimacy. In other words, they're horny and want to get it on! Remember the old Bad Company song, *"Feel Like Makin' Love"*? That's basically the soundtrack for both partners in the first year of a relationship.

After about a year, though, the woman's theme song begins to sound more like Beyonce's *"Single Ladies (Put a Ring on It)."* Typically, women's brain chemistry moves away from the perpetual horniness driven by testosterone, serotonin, dopamine, norepinephrine and epinephrine, towards a calmer, oxytocin-based state, which is marked by the desire for bonding and partnership. Ironically, sex is a big part of bonding in a relationship, especially for men. (Here's something interesting: after their partner has a baby, oxytocin levels rise in men, so they don't get the urge to kill the offspring, which is common in some species.)

So as a relationship progresses, women's brain chemistry tend to move away from spontaneous sexual drive into a more sexually neutral state. They're not feeling the same level of desire to initiate sex, but they still want the bonding. Biologically, men like the chase and the game, and lots of sex keeps them interested and bonded to their partner. (Obviously, I'm generalizing in this explanation to illustrate what's going on biologically.)

So, if women's biological makeup were more strategically oriented (or followed the "no sex before marriage" rule espoused in most religions and self-help books like *The Rules*) we'd begin in a sexually neutral state and after about a year, move into the horniness stage to get what our minds/bodies are telling us we want! Biologically, women are programmed in the opposite way to men, and that's why so many relationships tend to crumble around the 1-2 year mark. As the relationship goes on, sex may become less and less frequent. Women are left wondering why their partner doesn't want to settle down after the excitement of that first year dies down. Biologically speaking, we're at cross purposes.

Back to Melissa. Her doctor wasn't aware of these natural sexual changes and focused on treating what appeared to be depression. Antidepressants, like oral birth control pills, also pump out serum binding hormone globulin, or SHBG. This binds up free testosterone, which is required for sexual motivation, desire, clitoral sensitivity, and the potential for orgasm. Melissa went to the doctor to get help with her waning sex drive, and the doctor unknowingly made it much, much worse. Doctors today, thanks to lack of training and undue influence from Big Pharma, are in the habit of prescribing antidepressants for a cornucopia of so-called symptoms in women that do not indicate clinical depression. I have one patient who was actually prescribed the drug Lexapro® to curb her vivid dreams!

In addition, there's a HUGE gender bias in treating depression-like symptoms. A male patient is far more likely to undergo a battery of tests to rule out any physical causes, while a woman is more likely to get handed a prescription for antidepressants. Also, medical school training is limited in terms of women's health. Medical students are taught to order certain tests, but not others, and they look at results in a linear fashion, when they should be examining them holistically and in conjunction with other tests and the patient's symptoms.

A caveat: Pills like Wellbutrin® and Effexor® cause fewer sexual side effects because they have a norepinephrine component, versus the majority of others, which are mainly serotonin-based. Norepinephrine has fewer sexual side effects, but in higher doses, it can cause the same issues. But Melissa is on Prozac. She's not just in a sexually neutral state; the drug is killing her sex drive altogether. Talk about a really vicious circle!

Feeling worse than ever, Melissa confides in a close friend, who refers her to me. I wean her off of the pills as fast as I can. However, and I can't stress this enough: It is important that you *never go off of antidepressants without talking to your doctor, and never, ever go off of them cold turkey.* This can be very dangerous.

Not only do antidepressants cause low libido; they also set up women for extensive health problems down the road due to the loss of testosterone. I give Melissa a jumpstart with a pellet of testosterone, and monitor her over time until her levels go back to normal. Women like Melissa can feel better as soon as the first month, but it's not uncommon to have to fiddle with the dosage for the first couple of months to get it right.

Within three months, Melissa's feelings for Eduardo warmed up again. While she's not exactly a randy newlywed, her overall mood and attitude have improved, and she has a sex drive again. Eduardo was immediately receptive – he takes her on romantic weekend trips more often, and they have a lot more fun together, both during the day and between the sheets.

CHAPTER SIX

HAVE YOU SEEN MY YOUTH? I'M SURE IT'S AROUND HERE SOMEWHERE: ESTROGEN DEFICIENCY IN THE 40S

"Not only is my short-term memory horrible, but so is my short-term memory." — *someecards.com*

The early- to mid-40s is when most women start to feel major changes due to hormone deficiency. Remember when we talked about the stages of menopause? Karen, 45, is smack dab in the middle of the second stage of perimenopause: estrogen deficiency.

This is when things really get ugly for most women, and Karen's symptoms are common. First, she's having difficulty sleeping. She used to have night sweats on occasion, but now they wake her up a few times a week. Sometimes she soaks through her pajamas and sheets, and has to get up and change her clothes and bedding. The lack of rest worsens her mood swings during the day, which are already pretty bad – she vacillates between being excessively crabby or totally apathetic. She lets minor irritations bother her and thinks other people are "stupid," so she lashes out at the smallest provocation. A waitress making an honest mistake on the bill or a person with 16 items in the 15-items-or-less line at the grocery store can push her over the edge. She has crying jags for no reason. Occasionally, panic attacks set in. With all that's going on, she's left wondering what's wrong with her.

The lack of sleep does nothing to improve Karen's memory. She has trouble remembering simple things, such as why she entered a room or where she put her keys. Her grandmother has Alzheimer's and she gets worried she's on the same road. Another concern: frequent heart palpitations, which make her wonder if she has a heart condition.

Karen gets migraines often, and has more general aches and pains. She feels less attractive lately due to the "middle age spread" that widens her midsection more each year. She gets regular exercise, but it's a struggle because she's always tired, and it's not helping her curb her weight issues. Her weight and poor body image causes her considerable emotional distress. She doesn't feel like she's attractive to her husband, James, and she has started wearing baggy, shapeless clothes to cover her widening waistline. Her libido has sunk to nonexistent levels.

In Karen's mind, she's still a fun-loving 26-year-old, and it frustrates her that she feels and looks older all. James loves her, but wonders how this frumpy middle-aged lady took the place of his cute, bubbly wife. Karen decides to seek medical help.

The first doctor Karen sees diagnoses her with fibromyalgia. There's no truly effective test for it; it's mainly a diagnosis of omission. Doctors don't think about hormone deficiencies, or they don't realize the symptoms mimic testosterone, thyroid or vitamin D deficiencies. (Here's the kicker: Most women have all three by the time they come to see me, and no one has diagnosed any of them properly.)

"Dr. Uno" prescribes a sleeping pill, pain reliever, and antidepressant, and tells her to get more exercise to help her lose weight and help mitigate her aches and pains, since exercise kicks the body's natural endorphins into gear. For Karen's libido, the doctor tells her to schedule "date nights" with James so she can get in the right frame of mind for sex. But Karen is often too upset or too unmotivated to go to the gym, and often after the dinner-and-movie date nights, she's too exhausted to do anything in the sack besides sleep.

Karen continues to feel worse, so she gets a second opinion. She goes to another doctor ("Dr. Dos") and mentions a friend who experienced similar symptoms suggested that she might want to get her thyroid and hormones checked. Dr. Dos sees that Karen has a diagnosis of fibromyalgia from Dr. Uno and immediately labels her as a problem patient. (Doctors profile like this all the time – it wasn't just a funny situation that happened to Elaine on the TV show "Seinfeld.")

She tells Karen she's too young to have hormone issues, but in reality, Dr. Dos doesn't want Karen coming into the office over and over, monopolizing her time. She sends Karen to get her blood work done, mainly to prove her wrong and shut her up.

When the lab work comes back, Dr. Dos tells Karen it's normal. Based on her previous diagnosis of fibromyalgia (which by the way, many doctors think is psychosomatic) she suggests Karen might get some relief from a psychiatrist, Dr. Tres. He acknowledges Karen is a very unhappy woman and prescribes another antidepressant, which causes a downward spiral — even more testosterone deficiency — and makes everything worse.

Now Karen is angry. She feels miserable, she knows her doctors think she's crazy, and she wonders how she got to this point. She was always a stable, strong, energetic, hard-working person who built up her own small business — not a whiner or complainer. An unintended consequence of all of this is her insurance premiums went up. That certainly doesn't help. She's already stressed out about money because she's self-employed, and she has missed some lucrative opportunities because she's too tired or zoned out to work like she once did.

A friend of Karen's tells her about me, and invites her to one of my Hormonal Happy Hours. We regularly host informal events with cocktails and appetizers, where we can share stories, present quality information about hormone health, and dispel myths about hormone replacement therapy. Most importantly, we help women understand that much of what they are feeling usually indicates they have a hormonal deficiency
– not fibromyalgia or depression – and that their symptoms and deficiency can be easily treated. Karen makes an appointment to see me.

I test Karen's hormone levels and do a full medical screen. We find out her testosterone is almost nonexistent. A normal level is around 100-150 when properly replaced, and hers was 5. Her overall estrogen and estradiol levels looked normal, but I take a closer look at the follicle stimulating hormone (FSH), which reveals how Karen's brain is responding to the estradiol being produced by her ovaries. Each of us is different. FSH levels rise and fall corresponding to the different phases of our cycle. The particular phase of our cycle will determine whether the FSH level measured on that day is normal for us. At this point in time, I expect Karen's FSH levels to be elevated, and I'm right.

As I've mentioned before, it's important to listen to the patient and not just look at numbers, which are only useful in conjunction with listening to the patient's symptoms. Both estrogen and FSH levels might be normal on the day of the test, but become erratic at other times during the month. At this point, given the severity of Karen's symptoms, FSH is typically trending upward based on her stage of perimenopause. FSH levels rise as ovarian function decreases, because FSH is trying to whip the ovaries into producing more estrogen. But if the ovary is slowing down or heading toward retirement, it's like beating a dead horse.

In addition, I notice Karen is hypothyroid based on her symptoms and clinical exam. First, she tells me she's fatigued, has gained weight, is intolerant of the cold, and has constipation and muscle aches and pains. She's most upset about the fatigue, because it's causing her to lose both productivity and potential earnings. But she's also pretty unhappy with the weight gain. Karen has clinical signs that clearly indicate she is hypothyroid, including slow heart rate, dry skin, thinning hair, slow reflexes, swelling of hands and feet, and swelling of thyroid in the front of the neck.

Lastly, I do a more exhaustive thyroid panel. Most doctors just check the thyroid stimulating hormone (TSH), and there's a wide spectrum of "normal" when reading this test. What may be normal for one patient is too low or too high for another. While a patient may be in average range, we're looking for optimal function. Working together, we can pinpoint their optimal range and get patients to the perfect level for them – and that's the one where they are feeling their best.

TSH levels also will appear more normal if a patient has lower testosterone, so it can be unreliable. It's important we also look at free T4, free T3, and reverse T3. Thyroid makes T4, but it's an inactive hormone. It has to convert to T3. A decoy molecule called reverse T3 does nothing but block the ability of free T3 to get to the receptors. Birth control pills, antidepressants and other medications, and adrenal problems are the most common reasons the body produces too much reverse T3. So we need to really delve into the entire thyroid panel — just looking at TSH is not enough.

Karen has been on and off oral birth control pills since she was in her twenties, and we already know that birth control pills and oral estrogens affect thyroid levels. In addition to increasing sex hormone-binding globulin (SHBG), the thyroid binding globulin (TBG) also goes up. It increases reverse T3 (a decoy) and lowers free T3, the active thyroid molecule. Labs will show the thyroid is functioning normally because doctors usually only check TSH — the brain hormone that goes up when the brain is not happy — and T4. But if we check T3 and reverse T3, it will show the active hormone molecule is bound up by the thyroid binding globulin, and probably will show more reverse T3, which is the decoy. Patients might make enough T4, but because it's bound up, the body can't use it. As we've already established, it's an all-too common problem for women on the Pill.

Gradually and safely, Karen is weaned off of her antidepressants and other medications. She starts HRT and eventually reconnects with that 26-year-old inside of her. She sleeps better, isn't moody, has more energy, and no longer feels like she's losing her looks. This motivates her to cut out snacking and binge eating, and start going for regular walks. This, in turn, helps her drop a size, so she buys new, more stylish clothes.

James loves Karen's new outlook and appearance — and especially her newfound romantic feelings for him. They drive to the mountains to go hiking at least once a month (and stay in a remote cabin, where they reconnect on another level). Most importantly to James, date nights now end with something more exciting than a peck on the cheek.

The Trouble With Hysterectomies

Not all women follow the normal route into perimenopause. For a variety of medical reasons, women might have a hysterectomy, which wreaks havoc on hormone levels, even when the ovaries remain.

Take Karen's sister Heather, 40, for instance. Though she's younger than Karen, she's always had problems with uterine fibroids. She has very heavy periods and cramps, so her doctor recommends uterine ablation. This is usually an outpatient procedure that uses laser, heat, electricity, freezing, or microwave to destroy the uterine lining. It's supposed to lessen or stop the bleeding, and doctors often try it as a "first step" in lieu of a partial hysterectomy. It only has a 50-50 shot of working, and unfortunately for Heather, it didn't. She experienced ongoing bleeding and extreme cramping, so she opted for a hysterectomy that left her ovaries in place.

Doctors mistakenly believe removing the uterus but leaving the ovaries in place – commonly advised if a woman is in her thirties to forties – will maintain women's hormonal health until they go through menopause. Heather's doctor assured her she should have 10 to 15 more years of good hormonal health with her ovaries; keeping her bones strong and protecting against cardiovascular risk, high blood pressure, high cholesterol, heart attack and stroke.

However, even younger women who have their uterus removed while leaving the ovaries will experience a drop of 30 to 50 percent in their estrogen function. Almost all will develop testosterone deficiencies immediately. Here's why: the arteries that supply oxygen to the ovaries are clamped off during the surgery so the patient won't bleed as much, which damages the ovaries. In effect, the ovaries are experiencing "mini- strokes" due to the blood constriction. In addition, some of the arteries attached to uterus and ovaries are removed during the hysterectomy, which reduces blood flow to the ovaries permanently.

After Heather had her uterus removed, she wasn't bleeding or having periods – a relief to her, but it masked the fact that she was unknowingly in early stage perimenopause. She became depressed, started gaining weight and then became pre-diabetic, and saw a rise in blood pressure, all due to testosterone deficiencies. She got occasional hot flashes and felt warm most of the time, but couldn't tell if it related to her ovulation cycles, because she wasn't having periods. Her doctor chalked up her issues to "getting older" and recommended blood pressure medication.

Heather knew something more was wrong. A quick Internet search yielded a nationally respected website for health, but the information didn't make sense to her. It was confusing and contradictory. Heather confided in her sister about her health concerns, and Karen told her about hormone therapy and suggested she see me. I ran a full evaluation. Lab work showed Heather's testosterone was severely low. Although her FSH and estradiol levels were normal, indicating she has normal estrogen levels and can produce eggs; I knew she had low estrogen based on her symptoms of mild hot flashes and feeling warm. I also diagnosed her as hypothyroid — not surprising, because this runs in families, and Karen had the same issues.

For treatment, I decide to place a small supplemental dose of estrogen and a full replacement dose of testosterone in pellet form subcutaneously. I also prescribe Armour thyroid medication.

Five weeks later, I rechecked Heather's levels. As her hormone levels rose, she had experienced some mild acne breakouts. (Replenishing hormones can be akin to going through puberty again.) These minor issues didn't outweigh the benefits. Heather has more energy, her libido is back, her memory is sharper and the hot flashes and breakouts are gone. She feels like her old self again. And once her hormone levels were steady and balanced, her acne went away.

CHAPTER SEVEN

MENOPAUSE IS NO LAUGHING MATTER: ESTROGEN LOSS IN THE 50S

Menopause: the very word can strike fear into otherwise strong and confident women's hearts. Musicals make light of it; women laugh and share war stories about it; but in reality, it's a serious situation. The loss of estrogen doesn't just mean hot flashes — it means an almost certain loss of quality of life and the onset of debilitating diseases.

Let's look at Sue, 57, a normal post-menopausal woman who feels anything but normal. She feels less attractive now that her skin is aging. It has a yellow hue, and she's getting wrinkles and developing the "bulldog jowls" that are a telltale sign of getting older. She's creaky and croaky; she feels less limber and more decrepit each month. Her memory is so bad that she often can't recall why she entered a room or where she left her keys.

Sue and her husband, Jeff, used to love to travel. They have ridden bicycles in China, hiked the Andes in Peru and snorkeled in Fiji. Lately though, just the thought of a long plane ride tires her out. Worst of all, her sex life is nonexistent. She not only has no libido, but intercourse is actually painful. Her husband, Jeff, is disappointed that sex has dropped off, but he doesn't enjoy it if it hurts her. They resign themselves to the idea that because they're getting older, they're stuck being companions and that's all there is to it.

I'm here to tell you it doesn't have to be this way. Like most women, Sue doesn't understand everything happening to her body medically, and that her problems are due to estrogen and testosterone deficiencies. The loss of estrogen that accompanies menopause causes rapid acceleration of aging. Taut, healthy skin gives way to thin, wrinkled and sagging skin. During the first five years of menopause, women will lose about 30 percent of their skin collagen and 25 percent of body collagen due to lack of estrogen. This leads to a host of other issues in addition to just looking old. Think about it: all of the tissues and mucous membranes in the body are affected.

After menopause, mucus membranes begin to thin out and dry up, and we begin to experience vaginal dryness. In turn, mucus membranes in the sinuses and lungs also become thin and frail. This allows more allergens and infectious agents to enter our bodies through the dry, cracked layers and irritate our lungs and sinuses. Voila, we develop allergies! We also have more vision problems, because the dryness in the eyes changes the curvature of the lens. In addition to the tummy and breasts sagging, the loss of elasticity causes the bladder to fall, leading to occasional or regular incontinence.

Like 63 percent of post-menopausal women, Sue has sleep disturbances. She not only deals with hot flashes and night sweats, but also has to get up to use the bathroom in the middle of the night because she can't hold it until morning anymore. She has to wear a thick pad when she goes out because if she coughs or laughs too hard, urine leaks out. Laughing so hard that you pee your pants isn't so funny once it becomes a reality.

On top of everything else, the vagina that used to be like a lush forest has become a dry desert. Sue's vaginal tissues are dry and thin, and they crack and bleed, causing painful sex. Dryness allows bacteria to invade, leading to more vaginal infections. Sue gets more urinary tract infections, too, because the tissue around the urethral opening thins out and dries up, allowing bacteria to travel up the urethra.

Oh, but wait. It gets worse.

At this age, women begin developing chronic diseases such as high blood pressure, strokes and heart disease, in large part due to the lack of estrogen. With proper estrogen levels, arteries and veins are flexible and elastic. Without estrogen, it's like leaving a new garden hose out to bake in the sun. It gradually becomes dry, hard and inflexible. Without estrogen, the arteries become stiff and don't bend anymore. Instead, they crack. When this happens, platelets congregate on these cracks, developing into small scabs. These scabs can flake off and potentially cause heart attacks and strokes.

Sue isn't quite there yet, but she is now beginning to experience bone loss — another major health risk as we age. Estrogen prevents the body from losing bone, and testosterone actually builds bone. So as soon as a woman goes through menopause and doesn't have these hormones anymore, she experiences dramatic bone loss the first several years. This is what Sue is going through.

Osteopenia, or low bone mass, is the precursor to osteoporosis (severe bone loss). This is often a silent disease. We have to screen for it and monitor it. If we don't screen for osteoporosis, we don't catch it until a patient gets a fracture.

I have a questionnaire that patients fill out to help me assess a 10- year probability of fracture. If a patient's answers indicate that she has risk factors such as family history of fractures, low vitamin D or calcium intake as adults, long-term use of certain medications, smoking, or a very thin build, among other factors, we need to obtain a bone mineral density test to assess her current bone density and risk for fracture.

If a woman starts taking estrogen before completing menopause, she most likely won't have bone problems. But hormones help even post- menopausal women. The Women's Health Initiative study showed that even when women were on the worst hormone products, Premarin and Prempro, hip fractures decreased by 30 and 40 percent, respectively.

The best thing you can do for bones is Mother Nature's therapy: estrogen and testosterone. Estrogen prevents bone from breaking down and testosterone helps build bone. Many patients are dead set against hormones due to the media hoopla spawned by misreporting of the WHI study results, but when I tell them that without HRT they'll have to take medications to treat bone loss, they usually change their mind.

Moreover, some osteoporosis medications are safe and some are not. I currently only prescribe two: Atelvia and Forteo. I prefer to rebuild the bones via hormones, but if a patient refuses, those are my go-to drugs, because they won't do further harm, like one of the most commonly prescribed drugs — Fosamax. Although Fosamax is extremely popular, I knew it was dangerous years ago when I worked at Procter & Gamble. Most drugs are processed though the body and leave the body via the urine. Bone drugs actually latch onto bone and stay there up to 50 years per dose, as in the case of Fosamax. You might think that's a good thing, but not necessarily. If a drug works too well, it can actually harm the bones in the long run. How?

Our bones are living, breathing organisms. We get micro fractures — microscopic cracks in the bone — all the time, just from walking, jogging, dancing, jumping on a trampoline, and so on. These tiny cracks are constantly being repaired, or "remodeled." Cells in the body called osteoclasts eat out the bad bone, like Pac-Man, and other cells called osteoblasts repair it by layering in a soft substance that hardens — basically like Bondo for the bones. This combination is called a "remodeling cycle."

Before menopause, the number of osteoclast and osteoblast cells is about even. As we age, due to estrogen loss, the number of osteoblasts decreases. Fosamax kills the osteoclasts, which allows the osteoblasts to function, but it does its job so well that it also decreases osteoblasts. It shuts down both sides. Now those micro fractures aren't getting filled in. Because the lack of cells prevents the remodeling, in the long run, Fosamax makes the bones brittle and more prone to major fractures.

Atelvia, though it's in the same class as Fosamax, allows for bone to heal and remodel. Forteo is in another class, called an anabolic agent, which allows bone to build and increases osteoblastic activity. I use this more expensive drug, which is injected daily, if a patient can't tolerate Atelvia (some get bad heartburn or muscles aches and pains on these drugs). Women on hormones, however, shouldn't have to take any medications. One study showed women taking combined estrogen and progestin with 1200 milligrams of calcium daily had a 60 percent lower risk of hip fracture.

In the United States, 10 million people have osteoporosis, and 90 percent of them are women. Among White American women, who are at a higher risk, 37 to 50 percent will have low bone mass or osteopenia, and 13 to 18 percent will suffer from osteoporosis.

I can't emphasize how important it is to maintain bone strength. After breaking a hip, the likelihood of death within the next year goes up 20 percent. That patient will also be 25 percent more likely to need long- term care. In addition to the pain, discomfort, and expense, 50 percent never regain functionality, and many end up in nursing homes. Or, if a patient can't afford care, family members end up with the job, which often hurts them financially and emotionally. It's estimated that osteoporosis-related fractures effect 25 million people each year and cost $16.9 billion annually.

By not taking HRT, you're setting yourself up not only for not feeling well and possibly having brittle bones, but also for developing a host of chronic illnesses. I regularly see women who are on 10 to 20 medications for issues including high blood pressure, bone loss, sleep problems, yeast infections, urinary incontinence, high cholesterol and coronary artery disease. Without HRT, post-menopausal women feel like they're aging overnight. They aren't old, but they feel and look old.

There is hope. HRT works wonders in post-menopausal women by restoring the body's ability to bring back collagen, so it's like getting a mini-facelift. I can tell you if a woman is on estrogen or not just by looking at the condition of her skin. It not only tightens the external skin, but now vaginal tissues will repair, the bladder will lift, and the arteries regain flexibility; so blood pressure goes down. It reverses the damage rather quickly. Women on HRT also are better able to fight off debilitating illnesses.

No one will live forever, of course, but multiple studies suggest women on hormones live longer, and are definitely happier later in life. Estrogen decreases likelihood of colorectal cancer, invasive breast cancer, and heart disease. It protects against collagen loss in intervertebral discs. It helps women maintain a healthy body mass index and lowers the risk of diabetes. One study showed women who had used estrogen for more than 15 years had a 40 percent reduction in their overall mortality. Personally, I will be on hormones until the day I die. You will have to pry my hormones out of my cold, dead hands …

actually my cold, dead butt, as I use subcutaneous hormone pellets.

So what about Sue? I recommended HRT for her, which helps her regain bone mass, stops the incontinence and get restful sleep. Soon, her muscles aren't achy, and overall, she doesn't feel like an old lady anymore — or look like one.

Sue still has a uterus, so the appropriate treatment would include estrogen and testosterone pellets, and progesterone. I know that progesterone has two places in life, but there is some controversy. Prior to menopause, it helps prepare our bodies for pregnancy — very helpful to the growing baby, but on the down side, it also gives us those dreaded PMS symptoms. It makes us gain weight so we can feed a baby, makes us tired so we slow down enough to care for a baby in utero, and makes our uterine lining fluffy, so an egg can fall into it and develop comfortably.

After menopause, progesterone primarily has one role: to protect the uterus. Women who aren't getting estrogen don't need progesterone. But if we prescribe estrogen, we have to prescribe progesterone as well. Estrogen causes the uterine lining cells to grow — that desert becomes a lush forest again. Once we create the forest, the body releases it through periods, if you're premenopausal. But post menopausal, the uterine lining can get too thick and cause annoying spotting or bleeding. Even more worrisome, it can lead to endometrial cancer if the body doesn't shed it. Progesterone protects the lining from building up.

We can prescribe progesterone in two ways. The first mimics the premenopausal periods or cycles, by giving progesterone for 10 days a month and then stopping it. The second is to take progesterone nightly, which keeps the uterine cells from growing altogether. Each method has pros and cons. Cycling has advantages, but some women are very sensitive to the effects — it makes them have PMS symptoms like being bloated, tired, and crabby. We can limit exposure and lessen the likelihood or severity of symptoms by giving progesterone fewer days. Also, having a monthly "period" can increase metabolism a bit and help with weight loss.

However, most women can't bear the thought of continuing to have periods after menopause — ugh. So, they choose to take progesterone nightly. Using it helps them sleep and feel calmer. However, despite our best intentions at controlling bleeding, bioidentical progesterone sometimes causes intermittent bleeding and spotting because it's weaker and doesn't stabilize the uterus as well as the synthetics. If this becomes an issue, we need to consider switching to a synthetic version of the hormone, because it absorbs into the uterus better. Problem is, synthetics aren't as safe.

The two most common commercially available progestins are Aygestin (norethindrone) and Provera (medroxyprogesterone acetate), used in Prempro. Aygestin is the better synthetic version, because it doesn't have the overall adverse effects on cardiovascular and breast health as Provera does. I carefully explain the differences to my patients, so they can make an informed choice. If they don't want the bleeding and are reluctant to take synthetic progestins, then I have to take them off estrogen therapy. However, I can still give them testosterone, as it doesn't cause the uterine lining to grow. This alone helps with 50 to 80 percent of menopausal symptoms. Sue decides to deal with occasional spotting, and goes on nightly bio-identical progesterone along with estrogen and testosterone therapy.

After HRT, Jeff said Sue looks several years younger. He's always loved her no matter what, but now he's more attracted to her than ever; and ecstatic that they're active in the bedroom again. Sue also has more energy all day long and is eager to travel again, so she and Jeff have scheduled a "second honeymoon" trip to Italy. One of their goals – in addition to roaming around Rome, traipsing through vineyards in Tuscany, and seeing the Sistine Chapel – is to get busy in their 15th century hotel, giving a whole new meaning to the term "renaissance."

CHAPTER EIGHT

GIVING BACK WHAT MOTHER NATURE INTENDED US TO HAVE: TREATMENT OPTIONS

Now that you know all about the tricky business of hormones, you should know about the various treatment options, too.

The first thing you need to ask your doctor when you consider HRT is: Do you use synthetic or bio-identical hormones? It's absolutely essential for your health that you get bio-identical hormones.

Think of hormones as keys, and the receptors in your body as locks. Bio-identical hormones look and act exactly like the molecules made in your body. They are keys that fit perfectly into the locks, or receptors, because they mimic your own hormones identically. In fact, they should be called "bio-mimetic" hormones because they're like a twin of the hormone already in your body.

Synthetic hormones don't work exactly the same as the keys in your own body. In fact, they can block the lock and jam it. Some synthetics might turn the lock, but it could stick a bit or not "open the door" completely to the receptors.

One big misconception about bio-identical versus synthetic hormones is that ALL synthetic hormones come from pharmaceutical companies and ALL bio-identicals come from compounding labs. Not true!

Compounding pharmacies can make synthetic hormones, and pharmaceutical companies can make bio-identical hormones. Some synthetic hormones made by pharmaceutical firms are very dangerous for women and have been pulled from the market. Others, such as Estratest, Prempro and Provera, are still on the market, but nonetheless aren't good for you. They're not very close at all to the molecular structure of our human hormones. But pharmaceutical companies also make good, bio-identical hormones that are approved by the FDA. Examples of very good ones created in a lab are the Vivelle-Dot® patch, Estrace® cream and Prometrium® (an oral progesterone). These are completely bio-identical; they just happened to be made by a pharmaceutical company that figured out how to patent their version.

Now, we have to look at delivery systems. You can take hormones orally (via pills), sublingually (under the tongue), by creams or gels rubbed on the skin, via a patch you wear on the skin, or through a time- release pellet inserted under the skin. The differences (and potential dangers) include how they work and how well they work for the patient.

Pills: The advantage to pills is that they're relatively easy - just pop one in your mouth. However, there's a huge disadvantage. Hormones taken orally and processed through liver will increase clotting factors and risk for heart attack, stroke or blood clots. This is amplified for smokers, and becomes extremely dangerous. A lot of doctors freak out about prescribing hormones if a patient has a history of blood clots or smoking; however there's no increased risk as long as the hormones aren't being processed through the liver. But there's a big risk even for nonsmokers when they take hormones via a pill. Unless there's a truly compelling reason for doing so, I don't prescribe oral hormones.

Creams or gels: Typically these are rubbed into the thigh, bikini line or wrist once or twice a day. The advantages is that they're fairly affordable — $30-$70 a month, depending on if it's estrogen, testosterone or progesterone alone, or in combination. Disadvantages are many. They're in and out of your system in a day, so if you forget to use it in the morning, you'll have symptoms by the afternoon or the next day, at the latest.

Creams can also take a while to rub in. They can be uncomfortable if it's hot. Gels can be sticky because they're alcohol or glycerin based. Some people, especially fair skinned and overweight people, don't absorb them well. Also, they deliver very erratic levels of hormone — at any point the level could be up to 50 percent too high or low for what your body needs. Overall, they're only about 30 percent effective.

Most importantly, they can be dangerous for kids, pets, or even spouses, and you must be extremely careful not to transfer them. For example, if a man comes in contact with estrogen, he can grow breasts or even begin to have PMS symptoms and hot flashes. A new patient of mine once told me she had a female dog that regularly licked her skin (likely because of the oils in her hormone creams) and the poor dog actually started to grow testicles!

Some women choose creams or gels due to cost. Others believe they're more "in control" of their hormone levels because they can choose when to apply them. But really, they're only in control of their symptoms, and they may not realize they're not getting high enough levels to help osteoporosis, blood pressure, heart problems, and all the other nasty issues that hormones can help prevent.

Troches: These work the same as creams and gels, but instead of rubbing them on the skin, the hormones are in a small gel capsule that's placed under the tongue, where it dissolves and is absorbed through the tissues. You take one or two per day. The advantage to troches is the relatively inexpensive cost (about the same as creams or gels), and they're safer than creams or gels for pets and other members of the family. Also, they're easily accessible.

Many women don't have a provider who understands the benefits of pellets, or maybe they're in an area where the nearest pellet provider is a long drive. Even though troches are made in compounding pharmacies, which aren't as common in less populated areas, you can get them via mail order. However, they deliver fairly erratic levels of hormones, with more ups and downs and side effects. Fits of rage, nightmares, and acne are more prevalent with troches, as well as creams and gels, because levels spike in the mid-afternoon. Taking half the dose in the morning and the other half in the afternoon can mitigate this, but it's still not ideal.

Patches: Good bio-identical estrogen options are the Climara®

and Vivelle-Dot® patches. These are what we call "matrix" delivery patches. They're infused with hormones that are slowly released into the skin. One advantage is that patches are often covered or partially covered by insurance companies, although it varies substantially, depending on the insurance company. With the patch, you will get more even levels, like a gentle roller coaster, versus spikes of hormone levels. Vivelle-Dot® is applied twice a week and Climara® patches are used weekly.

Yes, there are drawbacks. Some women can be allergic to the adhesive on the patch, so it's not a suitable option for them. However, the biggest issue is that most women will absorb the first 50 percent of hormones in the first 24 hours, and these are metabolized quickly. Your body will take what it needs and then it may not get enough, which can lead to hot flashes by the second day. Depending on which patch you're prescribed, you can have up to five days to go until your next patch. Also, with the patch you can only get estrogen, not testosterone, so again you only get half of the hormone equation.

We've already seen that the FDA — in a ridiculous decision not even remotely based on science — hasn't approved the testosterone patch for women. So if you use an estrogen patch, you must supplement testosterone with cream, gel or troches. Finally, if you're very active, sweat a lot or use hot tubs, the patches will often fall off.

There is one really good use for patches: The infusion of estrogen helps control menstrual migraines in women of any age. I prescribe them for patients who experience menstrual migraines for use when they're taking their placebo birth control pills on their "week off."

Pellets: These, in my opinion, are the gold standard. They're a little smaller than a grain of rice, and are inserted half an inch under the skin of the buttocks. First, we inject the skin to numb it, make a little cut in the skin, push them in, and then bandage it. The area is usually sore for a few days, and we recommend leaving the bandage on for three days. Most women find it only mildly uncomfortable for a short time; some don't feel it at all.

Over the years, I have personally been on virtually every hormone product ever created. Bio-identical hormone pellets are physiologically the same as our own bodies' hormones, and they provide the best and most consistent delivery and results.

In most women, we typically insert them three to four times a year and they don't have to think about it beyond that — no rubbing on creams or gels; no taking troches every day; no levels spiking on a daily basis. The levels are smooth, controlled and based on the individual needs of the patient. Our job is to figure out the proper dose and intervals so women have a constantly even, steady rate of release.

Pellets come in doses that typically range from 6 to 50 milligrams for estrogen, with the average being 12.5 to 20 milligrams. The body starts to store estrogen, though, so you don't need to use as much as time goes on. A dose of testosterone tends to run from 12.5 to 200 milligrams, with the average dose for women in the 100 to 137.5 milligram range. We use higher doses because our bodies burn it faster than estrogen, and we don't store it in our fat like estrogen.

Two main mechanisms control the release of the hormones in the pellet: the heart rate and brain. How does the heart rate control the release? The pellets are placed under the skin and blood circulates around it, gradually dissolving it, kind of like licking a lollipop. More active people will burn off the pellets faster than sedentary people, and everyone burns more during active times or workouts than while sleeping.

How does the brain control the release? If it senses a deficiency, it will gobble up the pellets and pull the hormones into the bloodstream faster. Women tend to burn the pellets off fast at first, especially if their hormone levels are very low and the brain senses they're essentially "starving" for the hormones.

Problems with Pellets

I hear a lot of women say they feel like crap on pellets. They cry all the time, their breasts are bloated, they gain weight and their extremities swell. These are common indicators that they're getting too much estrogen and not enough testosterone (and that they need to get a new doctor). Too many doctors are expanding into this field without having proper training or even a basic understanding of female hormone physiology. They don't know what they are doing, so they give the wrong doses and make women feel worse. Many will only use estrogen with little or no testosterone to balance it. We've already established that too much estrogen and not enough testosterone is a huge problem.

It takes a long time to burn out excess estrogen – in fact, it can take up to a year to get the levels back down. We carefully monitor patients and figure out the perfect dose for each person, keeping them at levels where they feel their best. Pellets bring as close as possible to the hormone levels Mother Nature once gave us.

Another, slighter disadvantage to pellets is that we can never be 100 percent certain if a dose is perfect until a patient gets them. The breakdown in my practice is this: 95 percent of the time, we get it right and patients feel great; 2.5 percent of the time, it's too low and they don't feel anything; 2.5 percent of the time, it's too high and they feel awful.

Women who get too much testosterone can experience anxiety, acne, and facial hair growth, and even rage. If the symptoms are significant, I can mitigate them with other medications, and the excess testosterone will be out of their system within a week. Symptoms of excessive estrogen, as we just listed, can usually be reduced within a couple of weeks and eliminated within a month. However, most side effects are mild, so we usually let them run their course, and the symptoms will subside naturally and usually go away within a week.

OK, there is one more disadvantage to pellets. They can be cost prohibitive, and a lot of practitioners don't accept insurance, so it's cash only. On average, pellets cost only about $100 to $200 more than gels and creams annually, but for people who are on a month-to-month income, it can be much easier to pay out in smaller amounts, so they opt for gels or creams.

Costs and Choosing the Right Provider

As awareness of hormone replacement therapy grows, there will always be practitioners who charge outrageous fees, whether or not they're any good at their job, let alone have proper training and knowledge. One group I know of charges $5,000 annually for pellets, and frankly, they're not worth it. A former mentor of mine charges patients anywhere from $3,000 to $5,000 for a three-hour initial consult, and because she is a highly respected women's health practitioner, her patients are willing to pay it; but the price is out of reach for most women.

With so many women desperate for help, I will caution that there are those who are "jumping into the game" and presenting themselves as experts, offering bio-identical or other types of hormone replacement therapies without proper training or any real understanding of the science behind it. Many of these types promote HRT as an aid to weight loss, libido enhancer or antiaging therapy to men and women, and they can be dangerous. Do your homework.

Faced with exorbitant prices, misinformation about HRT and the number of doctors who dismiss women's health concerns, too many women simply give up and become resigned to feeling like crap. DON'T. Knowledge is power. My goal is to educate and empower women so they don't have to go through the same struggles I did. I've made it my mission in life to change women's healthcare for the better. To this end, I have established The Hormone Health Institute: Executive Instruction for Medical Professionals, a training and consulting firm dedicated to educating my colleagues on HRT.

In my office, we accept most insurance plans, which usually cover consultations and office visits, minus deductibles and copays. Insurance usually covers blood work as well, but the push for coverage of hormone replacement therapy for women continues.

The real outrage? Although the quality of our lives and our health is at stake, virtually none of the insurers will cover HRT for women but many will cover for men. As the battle for equality continues, I will continue to speak out, fight and advocate on behalf of patients and women everywhere. I hope you'll join me.

CHAPTER NINE

YOUR HEALTH SURVIVAL GUIDE CHECKLIST

Now that you're convinced (you are convinced, right?) that hormone replacement therapy is a good thing for the majority of women, there's a boatload of information you need before seeing a doctor about it. This chapter is the heart of the matter: Your survival guide checklist. I've already outlined treatment options, but now, I want to go over details and symptoms of various hormone deficiencies; what to look for in a doctor, questions to ask the doctor once you're in the office (including which lab tests to have done), how to know if you're getting the proper treatment, and red flags to look for before and during the initial consultation. I'll outline all of this in a "cheat sheet" you can use.

Let's start by reviewing the potential symptoms of various types of hormone deficiency. Remember, if you're experiencing many of these, you may have the deficiency, but it could be something more serious. Work with your doctor to make sure you get a full panel of lab work and a thorough clinical exam.

ESTROGEN DEFICIENCY CHECKLIST

❑ Hot flashes, night sweats ❑ Dry or sagging skin

❑ Insomnia (difficulty getting to sleep, staying asleep or both)

❑ Heart palpitations or irregular heart beat

❑ Weepy for no reason

❑ Foggy brain or memory loss ❑ Decrease in lubrication

❑ Vaginal dryness, often leading to painful sex

❑ Urine leakage or incontinence   ❑ Sagging breasts

❑ Skin crawling or itching   ❑ Loss of hair   ❑ Worsening allergies

❑ Changes in periods (too early or too late)

❑ Heavy periods with clots and severe cramping

❑ Recurrent yeast infections or urinary tract infections

❑ Food doesn't taste the same   ❑ Burning mouth or dry mouth

❑ Dry eyes or change in vision   ❑ Dry hair and nails

TESTOSTERONE DEFICIENCY CHECKLIST

❑ Joint and muscle aches and pains (often diagnosed as fibromyalgia)

❑ Fatigue   ❑ Forgetfulness   ❑ Depression   ❑ Weight gain

❑ Irritability and decreased ability to tolerate "stupidity" in others or cope with life

❑ Anxiety, panic, sudden sense of doom; onset or worsening of previous mood disorder

❑ Food coma (feeling tired or needing to sleep after eating)

❑ Sugar craving (self-explanatory)   ❑ Low libido

❑ Lack of endurance during workout or taking longer to recover

❑ Onset of, or worsening headaches, including migraines

❑ Irritable bowel syndrome, constipation or bloating

❑ Difficulty reaching orgasm (often requiring more stimulation or time)

LOW THYROID CHECKLIST

❑ Extreme fatigue   ❑ Family history of thyroid disorders

❑ Given birth in the last 9 months

❑ Difficulty with breastfeeding

- ❏ History of infertility or miscarriages ❏ Smoking history
- ❏ Carpal tunnel ❏ Anxiety or depression
- ❏ Muscle and joint aches and pains (fibromyalgia)
- ❏ Anxiety or depression ❏ Cold all the time ❏Weight gain
- ❏ Difficulty losing weight despite proper diet and exercise
- ❏ Abdominal distention/bloating ❏ Constipation
- ❏ Difficulty sleeping Shortness of breath ❏ Dry skin and hair
- ❏ Swelling of the hands and feet ❏ Feeling "puffy"
- ❏ Brain fog, difficulty concentrating or memory loss
- ❏ Hair loss or thinning, coming out in clumps ❏ Goiter
- ❏ Voice is hoarse or raspy ❏ Loss of eyebrows or eyelashes
- ❏ Irregular or heavy periods ❏ Difficulty swallowing
- ❏ Throat feels full or pressure/choking sensation in neck

ESTROGEN AND TESTOSTERONE CLINICAL INDICATORS

- ❏ Yellowish, dry, sagging skin ❏ Vaginal atrophy (thin and frail)
- ❏ High pH of the vaginal fluid/discharge ❏ Abnormal lipid findings
- ❏ Abnormal discharge of vagina, indicative of yeast or bacterial vaginosis
- ❏ Dry hair with brittle ends Flattening, drooping breasts
- ❏ Dry eyes, dry mouth with bleeding gums
- ❏ Loss of bone on bone density scan (DXA)
- ❏ Low estradiol and testosterone levels on labs
- ❏ High FSH levels ❏ Elevated blood pressure
- ❏ Elevated HA1c indicative of pre-diabetes or diabetes
- ❏ Elevated CRP (cardio-reactive protein levels)
- ❏ PVCs (premature ventricular contractions) or PACs (premature atrial contactions) on EKG (electrocardiogram)

❑ Overweight or obesity   ❑ Irregular heart rate

❑ Blood pressure irregularities   ❑ Low heartrate (bradycardia)

❑ Low temperature   ❑ Slowed reflexes   ❑ Brittle nails

❑ Swelling of the hands and feet (edema)   ❑ Dry skin

❑ Fullness of the face (puffy)   ❑ Coarse, brittle hair

❑ Loss of eyebrow hair on the outer edge

❑ Dry mucous membranes   ❑ Goiter   ❑ Abnormal lipids

❑ Cool to cold extremities, especially the fingers and toes

❑ Hoarse voice   ❑ Elevations in TSH   ❑ Low T4 or T3

❑ High Reverse T3   ❑ Low T3/reverse T3 ratio

How to Know if HRT is Right For You

1. You have symptoms consistent with the above deficiencies and they are affecting your quality of life.

2. You want to prevent chronic illness naturally.

3. You want to get off many of your current medications to treat cholesterol problems, high blood pressure, sleep troubles, etc.

4. You are willing to accept the media and conventional wisdom is wrong, and that you are making an informed choice.

5. You have been given proper choices for treatment, including bio-identical and non-oral hormones, and feel confident that you are getting good advice.

6. You are not undergoing any active treatment for breast cancer or other estrogen-stimulated cancer, such as reproductive cancers (uterine, ovarian, etc). You can consider testosterone replacement with your oncologist's support after your initial treatment course is finished and in remission (usually after one year). Estrogen replacement would not be prudent, even when you are in

remission, unless there are very compelling reasons, and you are far removed from the active cancer.

Questions You Need to Ask Your Doctor

1. Do you believe that hormone therapies are dangerous for women? Why?

2. Have you taken the time to properly learn the data? Are you willing to learn? (If the answer is no, RUN!)

3. Do you believe if I am still having my period on a regular basis that I cannot possibly have hormone deficiencies? Are labs not helpful until you stop having periods? (If the answer is yes, RUN!)

4. Do you think that taking antidepressants are the best course of treatment for my symptoms? (If yes, RUN!)

5. Will you consider my clinical signs and symptoms and use labs to confirm diagnosis, or will you rely solely on labs to make my diagnosis?

6. Are you going to order a full thyroid panel including TSH, total T4, free T3 and reverse T3, as well as a full hormone panel including testosterone, estradiol, and FSH?

7. Do you have experience in interpreting these tests? If not, do you know someone to refer me to? Are you willing to learn?

8. When you treat hormone imbalance, do you use bio-identical hormones and non-oral treatments?

Red Flags to Look For at the Doctor's Office

1. Says you're too young to have hormone deficiencies.

2. Wants to put you on antidepressants prior to addressing hormonal concerns.

3. Doctor or staff is rude, condescending or apathetic.

4. Doctor spends only 10 minutes with you, and does not

allow you to talk or express your concerns or thoughts.

5. Tells you that you only need more rest, less stress and more exercise.

6. Acts impatient or patronizing, especially when you are expressing what you may have learned through your own research efforts.

7. Does not understand hormone labs and which ones are the proper ones to order.

8. Expresses anger or disappointment in your desire to obtain a second opinion, or request to send you to a hormonal expert.

9. Asks the same questions over and over again on multiple visits, appearing to have forgotten all your previous concerns or health history.

10. Upon your request for a different drug or treatment, the doctor refuses to prescribe it and won't explain why.

11. The doctor states, "There is no data to support it" in regards to something you're asking about or showing them. It simply means he or she isn't aware of the data, or doesn't know the data. If they don't know the data, ask them to refer you to someone who understands it.

Most important takeaway: You must be an advocate for your health. Ask questions, and don't be afraid to fire your doctor if he/she doesn't understand or want to understand your issues. YOU are in charge.

CHAPTER TEN

SUCCESS STORIES: BACK IN THE SADDLE AGAIN!

One of the most rewarding aspects of my practice is knowing I'm helping women improve their quality of life both in the short- and long-term, and I get to do it on a daily basis. Patients constantly thank me, but when they feel better, their spouses and families thank me, too! Here are a few letters from my patient's husbands testifying to the power of good hormone health.

Back to Her Old (New) Self

Dear Dr. DeRosa,

I have been meaning to thank you for giving me back my happy, sexy wife. I cannot thank you enough. We are now back to the way we used to be. Cindy is 10 years older then me but I never felt the age difference until she started having menopausal symptoms.

She knew something was wrong; she was gaining weight even though she watched what she ate, and she started waking up in the middle of the night with hot flashes and night sweats. She kept going to different doctors, but all the doctors would do is tell her she was depressed and give her anti-depressants, which had their own side effects. Some did offer HRT meds, but we were both worried about her taking them because my mother was on HRT for years, and they believe it contributed to her breast cancer.

I came home from work one day about two years ago, and she said; "You have to watch this." It was an Oprah show on hormone replacement therapy and bio-identical therapy. Everything they were talking about was exactly what she was dealing with. We were living in Ohio at the time, and she searched and only found one doctor 50 miles away that charged $380 for her initial appointment, and none of the visits would be covered by our health care coverage.

We planned on moving to Phoenix last year, and just before we made the move, she lost her eldest son from a previous marriage. Obviously, this was a tough time for all of us, but especially for her when she was already not herself. She would cry all of the time and had to force herself to get out of bed in the morning. She is one of the strongest women I know, but she couldn't get over the loss.

She met a lady named Nancy who raved about you, saying that you had turned her life around. She suggested my wife make an appointment, which she did in January 2012. You diagnosed her with underactive thyroid and showed her how her hormone levels were way out of whack. You worked with her to get her levels back to normal, and here it is — August 2012 — and she is back to her old self. She is now able to actually start dealing with her grief. She is happy again, sleeps through the night, actually wants sex and even initiates it now, and we feel close again. She is back to her fighting weight and feeling sexy again and no longer has to deal with hot flashes or night sweats. She tells everyone she knows how wonderful she feels.

I cannot tell you what this has meant to me. You have given me back my wife, the woman I fell in love with, and I cannot thank you enough.

Martin Quinn

I Can't Keep Up

Dear Dr. DeRosa,

Please STOP treating my wife — I can't keep up — she doesn't let me get my rest! But it's been something else in our sexual relationship, after being married for 21 years and the aftermath of two grown children (20 and 19 years old). I don't know how to express my gratitude and begin to tell you how things have turned around.

She is more upbeat and has more energy than before. In the past, after having dinner and watching a little TV, she would go straight to bed and fall asleep early, leaving me with no play time (if you know what I mean).

I have to admit that at times, I need those days back. It truly has been a big change. I can't thank you enough. It's better than winning the lottery. Can you please call ME for an appointment!

Mario P Age: 43
Phoenix, AZ

Drugs, Sex and Rock-n-Roll
(OK. Maybe not the ROCK-n-ROLL)

Hormone replacement therapy saved our marriage and our sex life. My wife and I have been married for 28 years and I truly thought my days of great sex and calm emotions in our relationship were long gone. Don't get me wrong, I really love my wife, but at times I felt like at any moment she might "BLOW" for no apparent reason. The littlest thing would set her off. I was constantly walking on eggshells. As she approached menopause, her hormones were crazy. One minute she would be happy and carefree and the next minute she was, how can I say this politely, "a little CRANKY." Intimacy was elusive, at best. She was not interested in sex and our relationship was starting to suffer.

A friend told her about hormone replacement therapy, so she scheduled a consult with DeRosa Medical. They conducted a comprehensive hormone panel, checked her thyroid, vitamin B12 and D3 levels. They found that her hormones were way out of whack. The imbalance in her hormones made her body "angry" (hence the erratic emotions), and the lack of D3 and B12 made her energy levels low. The under-production of her thyroid also made weight loss virtually impossible.

DeRosa Medical designed a treatment plan, and I can happily say that after all her levels were brought back to normal, she is a different person. The impact on my life has been amazing! She is now focused on all aspects of her health, as well as that of her family. Her energy is seemingly boundless, her exercise regime impressive, and her demeanor positive and fun-loving. Her sex drive has returned ten fold and our SEX life is better than it was in our 20s and 30s.

Her transformation has motivated me to return to my exercise program, eat healthy, and, after much consideration, start testosterone therapy at DeRosa Medical as well.

Thank you for opening our eyes to the possibilities, and for helping us reinvigorate and rejuvenate our intimacy, our marriage, and our life!

Sincerely,
Brian S. (age 50) and wife (age
49) Scottsdale, AZ

She Wanted to Live

I remember when my wife lost hope. She would sleep for ten hours and wake up tired. She would struggle just to get through a normal day. Anxiety would shut her down. She would tell me that she felt like she was living in a bubble watching everyone else enjoy life, while she was trapped in her own private hell. Several times a week she would go sit in the front room of our house and stare out the window at the blue sky.

When she went to see her doctor, they told her she was just moody and depressed. They told her she was premenopausal, and sent her home with a bottle of antidepressants. For over ten years those pills kept her functioning. Those pills dampened her anxiety and depression, but they also dampened her joy. Those pills helped her deal with the weight on her shoulders, but caused her to gain weight. Those pills allowed her to have a comfortable existence. But she didn't just want to exist. She wanted to live.

For almost ten years she took antidepressants, and for ten years I told people that when it came to women's hormones, doctors were clueless. Like my wife, I had lost hope as well.

Finally, a lab tech at my wife's OB/GYN secretly referred her to your office. She was skeptical at first, but when she called your office, she started to believe. At her first visit, you listened. You understood. You took the time to explain. She came home with renewed hope. She was excited. I was anxious.

When she came back to review the blood work, you pointed to deficiencies with her thyroid, even though all of her previous doctors had tested her thyroid and found it in the normal range. You put her on a simple treatment plan that included sublingual B12, D3, and a low dose of thyroid medicine.

Within two weeks I started to see the woman I married emerging from the ten-year fog that had held her captive. She began to have more energy. She was capable of coping with stressful situations again. She laughed more. She smiled more. She lost weight. She was more intimate. She was beginning to live again.

I don't know all the science behind the progress, but I'm glad that I can now say that I know a doctor that understands women's hormones. Thanks for helping my wife live again.

Thanks for renewing our hope.

Brock B., married to Britt B. of Gilbert, AZ, 46

It Really Works!

My life and my wife's life have improved immensely because of DeRosa Medical. Nancy's headaches are virtually gone and her energy level is back to normal. I (we) could not be happier.

Before Nancy started bio-identical hormone therapy, we were literally forced to leave our home because the desert heat intensified the headaches. Now we run over to the California coast when we want to, not because of pain and discomfort. It is odd that people I talk to have doubts about this remedy, but I can attest that it really works!

Thanks,
Tom Myers

Life Before Pellets

Dorothy sat, she just sat, looking at the screen, whether it was the computer screen or TV screen, and she just sat.

Any conversation was short and to the point. Many questions I asked were quickly replied to, with no further discussion.

I would come home at night after working and try to talk to her while she was watching the TV. Her replies came in like torpedoes from the couch. Quick, curt replies meant to end any discussion.

I would compliment her, only to have the compliment rebuffed. She simply did not believe that she was pretty, but I was after something else. Which, in fact, I wasn't – I was just trying to reassure her she was pretty to me.

I knew she was having a hard time, but anything I tried to do was just discarded. This didn't go on for just weeks or months, but years.

One day when I was working at my pharmacy, I had a patient come in that talked about her new doctor. She was really excited about this doctor that actually took time, had extensive blood work done, and kept working with her till an answer was found for her problem. I have known this patient for years, and you could tell a difference in her overall health and mental state. She gave me Dr. DeRosa's card and I took it home to my wife.

It just sat there. It sat there for several months. Then my daughter announced she was pregnant. My wife decided she could not be a good grandmother in her present health status.

She picked up the card and called one morning. She made it clear she needed a doctor who was going to actually spend the time and effort to work with her, to get her health problems resolved. She didn't need another doctor who would just tell her to do something and leave the room.

Dr. DeRosa took extensive blood work before her first visit. The visit didn't last minutes, but was much longer. Dorothy started the hormone pellet implants, along with the other medications that where prescribed. She "bought into" Dr. DeRosa's recommendations because she believed that Dr. DeRosa had an answer for her concerns, and took the necessary time to address those concerns.

That was a year ago. Since then, she has dropped 15 percent of her weight. She is active, happy, and engaged in her life. We take trips together; she is working at a job she really likes.

We do things together! We can tease and be playful with each other.

Wow! She got her life back, and with that I got my wife, sweetheart and best friend back, too.

The whole family teases that this is the new 2.0 and no one wants the 1.0 back, ever. Her friends tell me how much happier she is and how much better she looks. They credit it with her finding a job she likes.

I know differently, and she can explain it to them if she wishes.

In the meantime, I will enjoy this new life I have found with my wife and will keep recommending Dr. DeRosa to those who come in to my pharmacy asking if I know a good doctor.

Kirk Jackson

You Have a Choice!

You don't have to accept all the changes that can occur in growing older. I am 66 and my wife is 64 years old.

Far too often, we just simply accept all the changes a body goes through as we age. The loss of energy; fatigue that happens to most, can often be off set or postponed thru exercise … we all know that. However, we seem to accept as inevitable, our loss of interest in intimacy and sex. For women it is often even more complicated, with symptoms of hot flashes, night sweats, etc.

The reality is that that is not an inevitability … it can be managed. My wife and I have learned and enjoyed the benefits of hormone replacement that the DeRosa Medical group can offer. It changed our life, and our perspective on life. Beyond the important physical changes that the treatments provide, I think the larger impact has been the mental/perspective life changes that accompanied the changes.

Have you ever reflected on going back in life to redo high school or college only to realize that "only if I could do it with my current mind and knowledge base"? Well … now you can possibly do that in some aspects of your personal life.

The hormone replacement treatments brought back the passion and sexual energy that had been ebbing away from our personal relationship. The treatments provided the ability to regain the energy and the sexual interest that had existed years ago, but it is now coupled with the additional years of knowledge in how to better enjoy my partner. It has been an incredibly satisfying experience and opportunity.

My wife and I have truly been better able to enjoy the intimacy and have more time to have fun with all of it … much more so than when we were younger. When we were younger, we were all going through the learning phases of marriage and distracted by the activities of trying to survive in the business world and raising a family. Sex and intimacy were things you tried to fit in between what had to be done.

While my wife and I are both still working full time, we have learned how to keep a better balance between work and play … and with the kids gone, we have more time and space to enjoy each other, and even explore new horizons together comfortably. We have now been married for over 41 years … but we never enjoyed our time together more than we are now.

It may not happen exactly this way for everyone … but why wouldn't you try? The worse that happens is you just get better physically.

Name withheld by patient request.

You Want to Do What? Now? Again?

At age 70, we were beginning to think that the prospects for an active life, including an active sex life, were beginning to fade into the past. We were assaulted by many of the most common age related ailments: tiredness, long naps, decreased libido, arthritis, and for my wife, painful sex.

We were taking lots of pills, maybe too many – the best modern chemistry had to offer. We didn't think about natural hormone replacement, or understand the many ways in which hormones interact with other meds and impact our daily lives.

Then along came Dr. DeRosa. My wife's response to hormone therapy was miraculous. Her sense of wellbeing and her response to treatments for her back and other ailments was quick to follow. I can't be sure all of this was due to hormone therapy – this was not a controlled experiment, and other things were going on at the same time. But I doubt the shots in her spine were responsible for her increased enjoyment of sex and her libido. The impact of the testosterone therapy was immediate and striking. We were like teenagers!!!

The question now is whether I can develop the stamina to keep up with her. Dr. D – can you do something for me?

JG, Scottsdale, Arizona

CLOSING THOUGHTS AND STEPS YOU CAN TAKE TODAY

Women of all ages are being told every day that real, physical health problems are simply all in their heads. Now you have read the evidence and discovered what you've always known or suspected is true. Feeling awful is not all in your head, and it's' quite likely that your doctor (and many of your medications) is slowly killing you.

Women and doctors have been tricked into thinking that treatments for symptoms of menopause or hormone imbalances put women and their health at risk when nothing could be further from the truth. Basic hormone deficiencies have the potential to destroy our health, our relationships and our quality of life. Can hormone replacement really help protect women (and men) against chronic illness? Yes.

Bio-identical HRT tricks Mother Nature into thinking our bodies are functioning just like they did in our prime. Good, balanced hormone levels help us feel and look our best. But it's not like the old commercials where Mother Nature is missing her taste buds, and mistakes margarine for butter every time. Remember those? She'd roar, "It's not nice to fool Mother Nature!" and throw in some lightning bolts and thunderclaps just to underscore her point.

I like to think she was angry because she was duped into eating some chemical crap she'd been told was just good as butter; when actually, it was slowly poisoning her. Fooling Mother Nature by using her own natural compounds is by far, a far better way to go, especially as women live longer lives.

Collectively, chronic diseases that are easily preventable and treatable through bio-identical HRT are putting a massive strain on our healthcare system. Each year, medication for these diseases and newly invented conditions are putting millions, no, make that billions of dollars into already deep pockets. And that's exactly why big pharma continues to work overtime to shut down our access to bio-identical hormones, medications like Armour thyroid and to compounding pharmacies. Once people find out that the symptoms and syndromes that close with "Ask your doctor about…." can often be improved or eliminated through bio-identical HRT, they won't need all the pills pushed on us through advertising and by uneducated doctors.

The fight for our lives, our health and our happiness continue to rage on more fronts that ever before. The barriers we are facing for access to proper healthcare have been put in place by power, money, misogyny and madness. Each day, legislators and lobbyists (largely male) are making decisions that will greatly impact women's health and their quality of life, and they haven't even asked us how we feel about it because, as always, it's about control and the bottom line.

Now that you understand how hormones really work in your body, and you know how to recognize when your hormones aren't balanced, you can use this new-found knowledge to ask the correct questions to find the right doctor to work with you:

1) **How to find a BHRT doctor with appropriate training?**

There are many organizations that offer physician training in hormonal and anti-aging medicine. The American Academy of Anti-Aging Medicine (A4M) is one of the world's best organizations and offers fellowships and board certifications in this area of medicine and is a highly regarded entity. You can search their website for professionals who specialize in anti-aging in your area or talk to your personal medical provider about attending some of their World Congresses or learn their course work. www.a4m.com

The Hormonal Health Institute: Executive Instruction for Medical Professionals, is an organization I have personally created to train and mentor clinicians who want to learn how to best care for women (and men) through proper management of BHRT. This high-level concierge training offers one-on-one training for providers who want highly personalized, hands-on training and coaching with on-going mentorship and counseling. www.drhotflash.com

Some providers have taken weekend courses and are jumping into BHRT treatment with very little education or just enough to be dangerous. This approach, although a good start, is most often not enough training to allow providers to truly understand the unique nuances of women's hormonal health as well as the need for long-term, on-going education and experience. It took me years, if not decades, to learn all that I have about hormones and how to appropriately treat patients. BHRT CANNOT be learned nor taught in a weekend. Buyers beware of those doctors who have taken this approach.

2) **How to Interview your doctor?**

Use the questions on page 95 as a guide to assess your doctor's willingness and ability to have an open-minded dialogue about BHRT and woman's health in general. Women are highly intuitive and you will get a sense about the meeting, if it is going well and if your doctor is receptive. If your doctor is receptive, I encourage you to share the following page with them to guide them to the right resources, so that they may also become an ambassador for women's hormonal health.

3) **What to bring to your appointments?**

Make a chart of your own labs as well as a list of all your symptoms as they relate to the hormone deficiency checklists. You may even pull out the lists in this book and bring them to your appointments. It is important to be organized to maximize your time with your doctor.

You are empowered to make informed choices about your health and wellness, and your life. As a woman and a doctor, I am fighting for YOU, and for the health and happiness of all women. We deserve better. It's why I wrote this book. It's your hormonal health survival guide. Keep it close. You're going to need it, my friend.

HANDOUT TO GIVE TO YOUR MEDICAL PROVIDER

Dear Doctor,

I have been experiencing hormone deficiency symptoms and have done a lot of research (and not with Dr. Google) toward that end. I just finished reading the book, "A Woman's Hormonal Health Survival Guide" by Dr. Angela DeRosa and learned many new things about hormones and how they are affecting my health and well-being.

I really want to explore optimizing my hormones and hope that you will help me with this endeavor.

I am hopeful that you will work with me on assessing my hormonal balance.

Do you have the proper training and understanding of this specialized area of medicine? If you don't, do you want to learn?

There are many organizations that offer physician training in hormonal and anti-aging medicine. The American Academy of Anti-Aging Medicine (A4M) is one of the world's best organizations and offers fellowships and board certifications in this area of medicine. They offer courses, fellowships and board certifications in this area of medicine. www.a4m.com

The Hormonal Health Institute: Executive Instruction for Medical Professionals is an organization, founded by the author of the book I mentioned above, that was created to train and mentor clinicians who want to learn how to best care for women (and men) through proper management of BHRT. This high-level concierge training offers one-on-one training for providers who want highly personalized, hands-on training and coaching with on-going mentorship and counseling. www.drhotflash.com
If you haven't read Dr. DeRosa's book, I encourage you to do so. Although it is written for patients like me, it stresses the importance of medical professionals not accepting conventional wisdom and learning the "true data" surrounding bio-identical hormone therapy.

Even if you are not comfortable assessing and treating me for hormonal optimization, I would ask you respect and support my journey.

Regards,

ABOUT THE AUTHOR

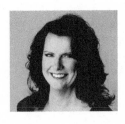 Dr. Angela DeRosa, DO, MBA, CPE, is a respected, internationally recognized authority on women's hormonal health who understands the range of health issues women face leading up to and during menopause. She experienced early menopause at age 35, with symptoms beginning in her mid-twenties, while she was attending medical school. In her quest to find out what was happening to her, it became clear that understanding, research and treatment for this critical phase of women's health was woefully inadequate.

Dr. DeRosa has more than 20 years' experience in the medical field, both on the pharmaceutical side and in clinical practice. She is the founder of DeRosa Medical, an Internal Medicine practice with offices in Scottsdale, Glendale, Chandler, and Sedona, Arizona. Dr. DeRosa is a member of the International Menopause Society, European Endocrine and Menopause Society, International Society for the Study Women's Sexual Health and a researcher on women's health issues. Dr. DeRosa is a Clinical Assistant Professor at Midwestern University, Arizona College of Osteopathic Medicine, and a Board Member and President for the Board of Trustees for the Arizona Osteopathic Medical Association.

The first edition of this book received wide attention from the public, media, and the medical community. In fact, Dr.DeRosa received an avalanche of requests from physicians across the country wanting to learn more. With that end in mind, Dr. DeRosa made the decision to be part of the solution and launched a hormonal health consultancy for physicians and medical professionals seeking training on bio-identical hormone replacement therapy. The new endeavor is called The Hormonal Health Institute: Executive Instruction for Medical Professionals (HHI). The Institute offers a variety of training formats and programs including live concierge-level one-one-one training in the physician's office, live and recorded webinars, self-paced digital classes, online group workshops, phone/email/Skype follow-up support, and peer support for physicians.

She lives in Scottsdale, Arizona.

RESOURCES (BOOKS)

Safe Hormones; Smart Women. Author: D. Lindsey
Berkson *North American Menopause Society,*
Menopause Practice: A Clinicians' Guide. 4th edition.

The Complete Book of Bone Health, Author: Diane L. Schneider, MD

Shmirshky; The Pursuit of Hormone Happiness, Author: Ellen Dolgen

Could It Be Perimenopause? Authors: Steven R. Goldstein, MD and Laurie Ashner

The Menopause Book, Authors: Pat Wingert and Barbara Kantrowitz

Living Well with Hypothryoidism, Author: Mary J. Shomon

Female Sexual Pain Disorders. Authors: Andrew T. Goldstein, Caroline F. Pukall, Irwin Goldstein

Clinical Gynecologic Endocrinology and Infertility. Authors: L. Speroff and F.A. Fritz 2004

The North American Menopause Society: Menopause Practice: A Clinicians' Guide 2007

What Your Doctor May Not Tell You About Hypothyroidism. Author: Kenneth Blanchard, MD

Sex Matters for Women: A Complete Guide to Taking Care of Your Sexual Health. Authors: Sallie Foley MSW, Sally A Kop, MSW and Dennis P Sugrue, PhD. 2002

It's My Ovaries, Stupid. Author: Elizabeth Vliet, MD

The Savvy Women's Guide to Testosterone. Author: Elizabeth Vliet, MD *Women, Weight and Hormones.* Author: Elizabeth Vliet, MD

Screaming to Be Heard. Author: Elizabeth Vliet, MD

The Savvy Women's Guide to PCOS (Polycystic Ovarian Syndrome). Author: Elizabeth Vliet, MD

Making Love the Way We Used To...or Better; Secrets to Satisfying Midlife Sexuality Author: Alan Altman, MD

Migraine Headaches, Hypothyroidism, and Fibromyalgia: Assessments and Holistic Approaches using Integrative Chiropractic, Naturopathic, Osteopathic and Functional Medicine. Author: Alex Vasquez

The Betrayal of American Women; Don't Throw Away Those Hormones So Quickly. Author: Alan Altman, MD

In Search of the Menopause Ranch. Author: Deborah Vaughn

The Secret Female Hormone: How Testosterone Replacement Can Change Your Life. Author: Kathy C. Maupin, MD, Brett Newcomb, MA, LPC

RECOMMENDED WEBSITES

DrHotFlash.com

EmpowHER.com

American Academy of Anti-Aging Medicine http://www.a4m.com

National Academy of Hypothyroidism www.nahypothyroidism.org

European Menopause and Andropause Society www.emas-membership.org/

North American Menopause Society (NAMS); www.menopause.org

The International Society for the Study of Women's SexualHealth.
www.isswsh.org

Center for Disease Control: http://www.cdc.gov

The International Menopause Society: www.imsociety.org

Society of Obstetricians and Gynecologists of Canada www.sogc.org

Summary of Hormone Therapy Findings for the International Menopause
Society: www.imsociety.org

Women's Health Initiative www.nhlbi.nih.gov/whi

Mary Shomon's Thyroid Info www.thyroid-info.com

American Association of Clinical Endocrinologists www.aace.com

American College of Obstetrics and Gynecology www.acog.org

Museum of Menstruation and Women's Health www.mum.org

Federal Drug Administration (FDA) www.fda.gov

RESEARCH REFERENCES

International Menopause Society; CLIMATERIC; The Women's Health Initiative-a Decade of Progress: Volume 15 number 3 June 2012

International Menopause Society Writing Group. Updated, IMS recommendations on postmenopausal hormone therapy and preventive strategies for midlife health. CLIMATERIC 2011; 14:302- 20

Davis, M. and R. Kroll. Testosterone improves sexual function in women not taking estrogen. The NAMS, First to Now. December 23, 2008; 359: 2005-2017

Haimov-Kochman, R. and D. Hochner-Celnikier. Are there second thoughts about the results of the WHI study? Acta Obstetricia et gynecologica Scandinavica 2006; 85(4) 387-393

Pines, A., DW Sturdee, et al. The heat of the WHI study; time for hormone policies to be revised. CLIMATERIC 2007 10; 267-269

Pines, A., DW Sturdee, et al. More data on hormone therapy and coronary heart disease. Comments on recent publications for the WHI and nurses health study. CLIMATERIC 2006; 9(2) 75-6

Pines, A., DW Sturdee, et al. HRT in the early menopause; Scientific evidence and common perceptions. CLIMATERIC 2008 11(4); 267-72

Shifren, JL, GD Braunstein et al. Transdermal testosterone treatment in women with impaired sexual function after oophorectomy. NEJM 200.; 343 (10) 682-8

Danforth, E. Jr. and A. Burger. "The role of thyroid hormones in the control of energy expenditure" Clinics in endocrinology and metabolism 13 (3) Nov 1984 581-95

Susan Davis, MD and Sonia Davison. Current perspectives on testosterone therapy for women. Menopausal Medicine. Volume 20, number 2 May 2012

Bernadette Biondi and Leonard Wartofsky, Combination treatment with T4 and T3: toward personalized replacement therapy in hypothyroidism. JECM July 2012;97 (7) 2256-2271

Writing group for the women's health initiative investigators, Risk and benefits of estrogen plus progestin in healthy postmenopausal women. JAMA 2002, 288; 321-33

Kolata G. Study is halted over rise seen in cancer risk; New York times, July 9th, 2002.

Rossouw JE, Prentice RL, Manson JE et al. Postmenopausal Hormone therapy and risk of cardiovascular disease by age and years since menopause. JAMA 2007; 297:1465-77

Gompel A, Santen RJ Hormone therapy and breast cancer risk 10 years after the WHI. CLIMATERIC 2012; 15:241-9

Burger HG, MacLennan, AH, Huang, K et al. Evidence based assessment of the impact of the WHI on women's health. CLIMATERIC 2012; 15:281-7

Brown, S. Shock, Terror and controversy, how the media reacted to the Women's Health Initiative. CLIMATERIC 2012;15:275-280

Lawrence Phillips MD and Robert Langer, MD, MPH Postmenopausal Hormone therapy: Critical reappraisal and united hypothesis. Postmenopausal Hormone Therapy Volume 83, No. 3, March 2005

The Women's Health Initiative Study Group. Effects of conjugated equine estrogen in postmenopausal women with hysterectomy: The Women's Health Initiative Randomized Controlled Trial. JAMA 2004; 291:1701–12.

Siris ES, Miller P, Barrett-Connor E, Faulkner K, Wehren L, Abbott TA, et al. Identification and fracture outcomes of undiagnosed low bone mineral density in postmenopausal women. JAMA 2001; 286:2815– 22.

Chen C-L, Weiss NS, Newcomb P, Barlow W, White E. Hormone replacement therapy in relation to breast cancer. JAMA 2002; 287:734–41.

Ursin G, Tseng C-C, Paganini-Hill A, Shelley E, Wan PC, Formenti S, et al. Does menopausal hormone replacement therapy interact with known factors to increase risk of breast cancer? Journal of Clinical Oncology 2002; 20:699–706.

Falkeborn M, Persson I, Adami HO, Bergstrom R, Eaker E, Lithell H, et al.
The risk of acute myocardial infarction after oestrogen and oestrogen-progestin replacement. British Journal of Obstetrics and Gynecology 1992; 99:821– 8.

Grodstein F, Stampfer MJ, Manson JE, Colditz GA, Willett WC, Rosner B, et al. Postmenopausal estrogen and progestin use and the risk of cardiovascular disease. New England Journal of Medicine 1996; 335:453– 61.

McNagny SE, Wenger NK. The controversy of postmenopausal hormone replacement therapy and cardiovascular risk reduction. In: Branch WT, Jr., Alexander RW, Schlant RC, Hurst JW, eds. Cardiology in primary care. New York: McGraw-Hill, 2003:253–64.

Adams MR, Register TC, Golden DL, Wagner JD, Williams JK. Medroxyprogesterone acetate antagonizes inhibitory effects of conjugated equine estrogens on coronary artery atherosclerosis. Arteriosclerosis Thrombosis Vascular Biology 1997; 17:217–21.

Cushman M, Legault C, Barrett-Connor E, Stefanick ML, Kessler C, Judd HL, et al. Effect of postmenopausal hormones on inflammation sensitive proteins: the Postmenopausal Estrogen/Progestin Interventions (PEPI) Study. Circulation 1999; 100:717–22.

When it Comes to Healthcare, Women Get Dismissed

A Woman's Hormonal Health Survival Guide: How to Prevent Your Doctor From Slowly Killing You takes a frank, tell-it-like-it-is look at the state of women's health. Common health conditions and diseases in women of all ages can often be traced to one root cause: hormone imbalances and deficiencies. and women can have them from the onset of puberty.

In the short term, these are a serious concern: sapping energy, causing mood disorders, memory problems and putting a damper on libido. In the long term, untreated hormone deficiencies are contributing factors in developing heart disease, diabetes, bone loss, obesity, cancer and other chronic health issues.

Find Out Why Women Are Suffering and Dying Needlessly Most medical professionals aren't trained to properly diagnose and treat hormonal deficiencies and don't understand their impact on overall health. And that's just the beginning! Underlying gender bias in American culture, medicine, and politics, combined with unbridled power and the very deep pockets of the pharmaceutical industry are all working against the best interests of women and their healthcare.

 Dr. Angela DeRosa began experiencing symptoms associated with menopause while still in medical school. By age 35. she reached menopause. Her quest to understand what was happening in her body launched her career specializing in women's health, with an emphasis on the importance of balanced hormones as a foundation for better health.
Today , Dr. DeRosa is an internationally recognized authority on women's hormonal health and has successfully treated thousands of patients.

DeRosa Media, LLC
11445 E. Via Linda
Dr.
Ste 2-206
Scottsdale, AZ 85259

Made in the USA
Coppell, TX
02 April 2023

15095462R00069